The Acupressure Handbook

Ancient Healing Techniques for Today's World

Mei Lin Zhang

Xspurts.com

A New Zealand Designed Product

Other Versions Available

Why limit yourself to just one format?

This book is now available in physical, digital, and audiobook options.

Choose the way you love to read and dive into the story today. You won't regret it!

Digital ISBN: 9781776968213
Physical ISBN: 9781776968206
Audio ISBN:

To obtain a different format of this book at a discounted price, please get in touch with us at:

http://isbn.xspurts.com/

Contents

Have Questions / Comments?

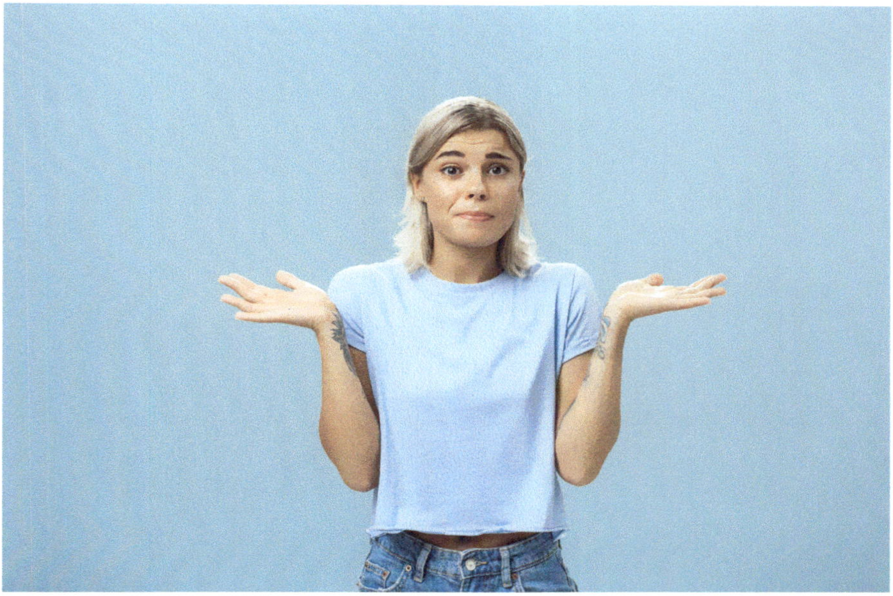

This book was designed to cover as much information as possible, but I know I have probably missed something, or some new amazing discovery has just come out.

If you notice something missing or have a question that I failed to answer, please get in touch and let me know. If I can, I will email you an answer and also update the book so others can also benefit from it.

Thanks For Being Awesome :)

Submit Your Questions / Comments At:

https://questions.xspurts.com

Get Free Stuff

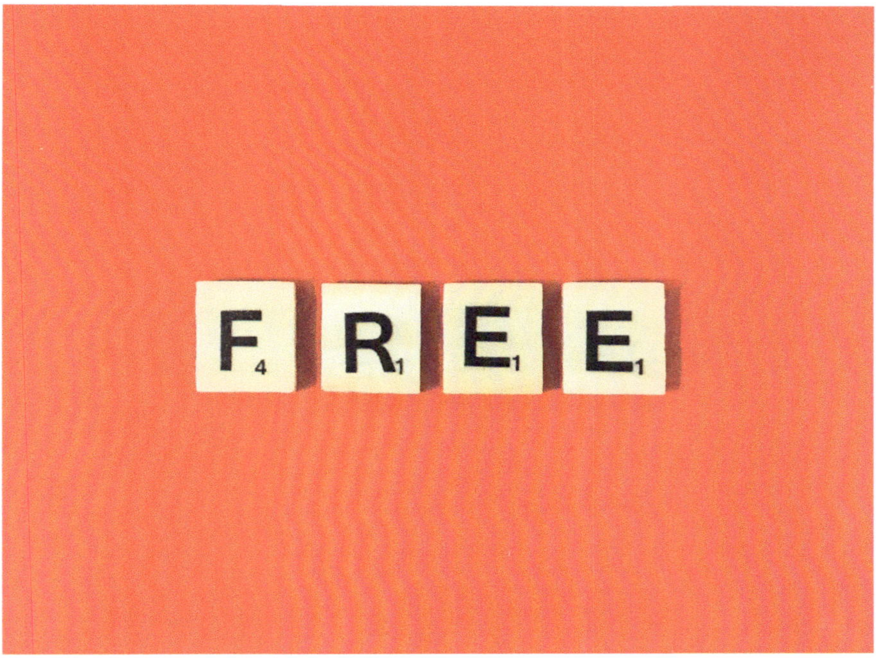

We love writing and have produced a huge number of books.

For being one of our amazing readers, we would love to offer you more books we have created, 100% free.

To claim this limited time special offer, simply go to the site below and enter your name and email address.

You will then receive loads (as we love our readers so much :) of our great books, content and audio direct to your email account, 100% free!

Get Loads of FREE Stuff at:

https://free.xspurts.com

Chapter One

Understanding Acupressure

Acupressure is an ancient Chinese therapy that involves applying pressure on specific points on the body to relieve pain, stimulate healing, and promote relaxation. It is based on the principles of Traditional Chinese Medicine (TCM), which views the body as a complex system of energy channels, or meridians, through which vital energy, or Qi, flows. When this energy is blocked or imbalanced, it can lead to various physical, emotional, and mental ailments.

Acupressure works by stimulating the body's self-healing mechanisms and restoring the balance of Qi. By applying pressure on specific points along the meridians, acupressure practitioners can activate the flow of Qi and remove any blockages or imbalances that may be causing pain or discomfort.

The acupressure points are located all over the body, from the head to the toes, and are associated with different organs, systems, and functions. For example, the point on the webbing between the thumb and index finger is known as the Hegu point and is associated with the large intestine meridian. Applying pressure on this point is said to relieve constipation, diarrhea, and other digestive problems.

Another example is the Zusanli point, located on the lower leg, which is associated with the stomach and spleen meridians. Stimulating this point is said to boost the digestive system, strengthen the immune system, and promote overall wellness.

Acupressure can be performed by a trained practitioner or by oneself. Self-acupressure techniques involve applying pressure on specific points with the fingers, thumbs, or other tools, such as acupressure balls or mats. One can also use acupressure in combination with other therapies, such as massage, acupuncture, or aromatherapy, to enhance their effects.

Acupressure has been used for thousands of years in China and other parts of Asia as a natural and effective way to relieve pain and promote healing. In recent years, it has gained popularity in the West as a complementary therapy for a wide range of conditions, from chronic pain and stress to anxiety and depression.

There is a growing body of scientific evidence supporting the effectiveness of acupressure in treating various health conditions. For example, a study published in the Journal of Acupuncture and Meridian Studies found that acupressure can significantly reduce menstrual pain in women.

Another study published in the Journal of Alternative and Complementary Medicine showed that acupressure can help reduce anxiety and improve sleep quality in patients with cancer.

Acupressure has also been found to be effective in relieving back pain, migraines, and arthritis pain. A meta-analysis of 16 randomized controlled trials found that acupressure can significantly reduce chronic low back pain.

Acupressure is generally considered safe when performed by a trained practitioner or when using self-acupressure techniques correctly. However, like any therapy, it may not be suitable for everyone and may cause side effects in some individuals, such as bruising, soreness, or dizziness.

It is important to consult with a healthcare provider before starting any new therapy, especially if you have a medical condition or are taking any medications.

History and Origins

Acupressure is an ancient healing technique that has been used for thousands of years in China and other parts of Asia. It is based on the principles of Traditional Chinese Medicine (TCM), which views the body as a complex system of energy channels, or meridians, through which vital energy, or Qi, flows. When this energy is blocked or imbalanced, it can lead to various physical, emotional, and mental ailments.

The origins of acupressure can be traced back to the Huangdi Neijing, or the Yellow Emperor's Classic of Internal Medicine, a text that dates back to the third century BCE. This text is considered one of the foundational texts of TCM and outlines the principles and practices of acupuncture, herbal medicine, and other traditional healing modalities.

According to the Huangdi Neijing, the body is divided into 12 main meridians, or energy channels, each of which is associated with a specific organ system and function. The meridians are also connected to the five elements of nature, including wood, fire, earth, metal, and water, which represent different aspects of the body and its functions.

The practice of acupressure involves applying pressure on specific points along the meridians to stimulate the flow of Qi and restore balance and harmony to the body. The pressure can be applied with the fingers, thumbs, palms, or other tools, such as acupressure balls or mats.

Over the centuries, acupressure has been used to treat a wide range of health conditions, from headaches and menstrual cramps to back pain and digestive disorders. It has also been used to promote relaxation, reduce stress, and enhance overall wellness.

Acupressure was introduced to Japan during the sixth century CE and became known as shiatsu, which means "finger pressure" in Japanese. Shiatsu is a form of acupressure that is still widely practiced today and is recognized as a separate form of therapy in Japan.

1. In the West, acupressure was largely unknown until the 20th century when it was introduced by Chinese immigrants and travelers. The first English-language book on acupressure, Acupressure: The Ancient Chinese Art of Healing, was published in 1971 by Dr. J.R. Worsley, an acupuncturist and practitioner of TCM.

Since then, acupressure has gained popularity in the West as a natural and effective way to complement conventional medical treatments and promote wellness. It has also been incorporated into various complementary and alternative medicine (CAM) practices, such as massage therapy, reflexology, and aromatherapy.

Today, acupressure is widely recognized as a safe and effective form of therapy for a wide range of health conditions. It is used by healthcare practitioners, massage therapists, and other wellness professionals around the world.

However, despite its widespread use and acceptance, acupressure continues to be controversial in some circles, with critics questioning its efficacy and safety. Some skeptics argue that acupressure is based on unfounded and unscientific theories and that its benefits are largely due to the placebo effect.

Nonetheless, scientific research has shown that acupressure can be an effective therapy for various health conditions. For example, a study published in the Journal of Pain and Symptom Management found that acupressure can significantly reduce nausea and vomiting in cancer patients undergoing chemotherapy.

Another study published in the Journal of Alternative and Complementary Medicine showed that acupressure can help reduce anxiety and improve sleep quality in patients with chronic obstructive pulmonary disease (COPD).

Research has also shown that acupressure can be an effective therapy for chronic pain, migraines, and other conditions. For example, a meta-analysis of 16 randomized controlled

The Principles of Acupressure

Acupressure is an ancient healing technique that involves applying pressure on specific points on the body to promote healing and wellness. It is based on the principles of Traditional Chinese Medicine (TCM), which views the body as a complex system of energy channels, or meridians, through which vital energy, or Qi, flows.

The principles of acupressure are rooted in the belief that the body has an innate ability to heal itself and maintain balance and harmony. When this balance is disrupted, it can lead to various physical, emotional, and mental ailments.

Acupressure works by stimulating the body's natural healing mechanisms and restoring balance and harmony to the body. It does this by activating the flow of Qi along the meridians and removing any blockages or imbalances that may be causing pain or discomfort.

There are several key principles of acupressure that guide its practice and application:

1. The Meridian System: According to TCM, the body is divided into 12 main meridians, or energy channels, each of which is associated with a specific organ system and function. The meridians are also connected to the five elements of nature, including wood, fire, earth, metal, and water, which represent different aspects of the body and its functions.

2. Qi: Qi is the vital energy that flows through the meridians and supports the body's functions. When Qi is blocked or imbalanced, it can lead to various health conditions. Acupressure works by stimulating the flow of Qi and restoring balance and harmony to the body.

3. Acupressure Points: The acupressure points are located all over the body and are associated with different organs, systems, and functions. By applying pressure on these points, acupressure practitioners can activate the flow of Qi and remove any blockages or imbalances that may be causing pain or discomfort.

4. Yin-Yang Balance: Yin and Yang are two opposing forces that are present in all things, including the body. In TCM, health is believed to be a state of balance between Yin and Yang. Acupressure works to restore this balance by removing any blockages or imbalances that may be disrupting the flow of Qi and creating disharmony.

5. Five Element Theory: The five elements of nature, including wood, fire, earth, metal, and water, are also associated with different aspects of the body and its functions. By understanding the relationships between the elements and the body, acupressure practitioners can better understand the underlying causes of various health conditions and tailor their treatments accordingly.

Acupressure can be performed by a trained practitioner or by oneself. Self-acupressure techniques involve applying pressure on specific points with the fingers, thumbs, or other tools, such as acupressure balls or mats.

One can also use acupressure in combination with other therapies, such as massage, acupuncture, or aromatherapy, to enhance their effects.

Acupressure has been used for thousands of years in China and other parts of Asia as a natural and effective way to relieve pain and promote healing. In recent years, it has gained popularity in the West as a complementary therapy for a wide range of conditions, from chronic pain and stress to anxiety and depression.

While there is a growing body of scientific evidence supporting the effectiveness of acupressure, more research is needed to fully understand its mechanisms of action and potential benefits. Nonetheless, acupressure is generally considered safe and can be a natural and effective way to complement conventional medical treatments and promote a healthier lifestyle.

Acupressure vs Acupuncture

Acupressure and acupuncture are both ancient healing techniques that originated in China and are based on the principles of Traditional Chinese Medicine (TCM). While both therapies involve stimulating specific points on the body to promote healing and wellness, there are some key differences between the two.

Acupressure is a therapy that involves applying pressure on specific points on the body to stimulate the flow of Qi and promote healing. This pressure can be applied with the fingers, thumbs, palms, or other tools, such as acupressure balls or mats. The pressure is applied for several seconds to several minutes, depending on the practitioner's technique and the client's condition.

Acupuncture, on the other hand, involves inserting thin needles into specific points on the body to stimulate the flow of Qi and promote healing.

The needles are left in place for several minutes to several hours, depending on the practitioner's technique and the client's condition. Acupuncture is often combined with other therapies, such as cupping, moxibustion, or electrical stimulation, to enhance its effects.

One of the main differences between acupressure and acupuncture is the way in which they stimulate the flow of Qi. Acupressure works by applying pressure on the surface of the skin, while acupuncture works by inserting needles into the skin. Both therapies can be effective in stimulating the flow of Qi and promoting healing, but some people may prefer one over the other depending on their personal preferences and health conditions.

Another difference between acupressure and acupuncture is the level of training required to practice each therapy. While acupressure can be learned and practiced by anyone, acupuncture requires specialized training and certification. Acupuncture needles must be inserted at precise depths and angles to be effective and safe, and improper insertion can lead to complications such as bleeding, infection, or nerve damage.

Acupressure, on the other hand, can be performed safely by anyone with basic knowledge of the acupressure points and techniques. However, it is important to note that improper technique or overuse of acupressure can also lead to complications, such as bruising, soreness, or dizziness.

Both acupressure and acupuncture have been used for thousands of years in China and other parts of Asia as natural and effective ways to promote healing and wellness. In recent years, they have gained popularity in the West as complementary therapies for a wide range of conditions, from chronic pain and stress to anxiety and depression.

While there is a growing body of scientific evidence supporting the effectiveness of both therapies, more research is needed to fully understand their mechanisms of action and potential benefits. Nonetheless, both therapies are generally considered safe and can be natural and effective ways to complement conventional medical treatments and promote a healthier lifestyle.

Chapter Two

The Science of Acupressure

Acupressure is an ancient healing technique that involves applying pressure on specific points on the body to promote healing and wellness. While acupressure has been used for thousands of years in China and other parts of Asia, the scientific understanding of how it works is still evolving.

One theory is that acupressure works by stimulating the release of endorphins, the body's natural painkillers. Endorphins are chemicals produced by the brain that bind to opiate receptors and can reduce pain, promote relaxation, and enhance mood.

Another theory is that acupressure works by stimulating the release of oxytocin, a hormone that promotes feelings of relaxation and well-being. Oxytocin is released by the brain in response to touch, and acupressure may enhance the release of oxytocin by stimulating the touch receptors in the skin.

Acupressure may also work by stimulating the flow of blood and oxygen to the affected areas, promoting healing and reducing pain and inflammation. By applying pressure on specific points, acupressure can increase circulation and promote the delivery of nutrients and oxygen to the tissues.

Some studies have also suggested that acupressure can modulate the autonomic nervous system, which controls many of the body's automatic functions, such as heart rate, blood pressure, and digestion. By stimulating specific points on the body, acupressure can affect the balance of the sympathetic and parasympathetic nervous systems and promote relaxation and healing.

Despite these theories and observations, the exact mechanisms of action of acupressure are still not fully understood. More research is needed to determine how acupressure works and to identify its potential benefits and limitations.

However, there is growing evidence that acupressure can be an effective therapy for various health conditions. For example, a systematic review of 35 randomized controlled trials found that acupressure can significantly reduce pain and anxiety in patients undergoing surgical procedures.

Another study published in the Journal of Alternative and Complementary Medicine found that acupressure can reduce nausea and vomiting in patients undergoing chemotherapy. The study also found that acupressure was effective in reducing the need for anti-nausea medications.

Acupressure has also been found to be effective in treating various types of pain, including chronic low back pain, headaches, and menstrual cramps. A meta-analysis of 16 randomized controlled trials found that acupressure can significantly reduce chronic low back pain.

In addition to its potential therapeutic benefits, acupressure is generally considered safe and can be practiced by anyone with basic knowledge of the acupressure points and techniques. However, it is important to note that improper technique or overuse of acupressure can also lead to complications, such as bruising, soreness, or dizziness.

It is also important to consult with a healthcare provider before starting any new therapy, especially if you have a medical condition or are taking any medications.

The Meridian System

The meridian system is one of the fundamental concepts of Traditional Chinese Medicine (TCM) and forms the basis of acupuncture, acupressure, and other traditional healing modalities. According to TCM, the meridian system consists of a network of energy channels, or pathways, that run throughout the body and are connected to the internal organs and physiological processes.

There are 12 main meridians in the body, each of which is associated with a specific organ system and function. The meridians are also connected to the five elements of nature, including wood, fire, earth, metal, and water, which represent different aspects of the body and its functions.

The meridian system is believed to be responsible for the flow of vital energy, or Qi, throughout the body. Qi is considered the life force that animates all living beings and supports the body's functions. When Qi is blocked or imbalanced, it can lead to various physical, emotional, and mental ailments.

The meridians are named according to their organ system and function, such as the Lung meridian, Liver meridian, and Stomach meridian. Each meridian is further divided into specific points, or acupoints, that correspond to different parts of the body and can be stimulated to promote healing and wellness.

The acupoints are located along the meridians and are identified by their specific location, such as the "Large Intestine 4" point, which is located on the hand between the thumb and index finger. Each acupoint has a specific function and can be stimulated through various techniques, such as acupuncture, acupressure, or moxibustion.

The meridian system is also connected to the body's circadian rhythm, with each meridian being most active during specific times of the day. For example, the Lung meridian is most active between 3-5am, while the Stomach meridian is most active between 7-9am.

According to TCM, the meridian system is also connected to the emotions and can be affected by emotional imbalances. For example, the Liver meridian is associated with anger and frustration, while the Lung meridian is associated with grief and sadness.

While the meridian system is a key concept in TCM, its existence and functions have been the subject of much debate and skepticism in the West. However, modern research has shown that the meridians and acupoints can be objectively measured and have distinct physiological and biochemical properties.

For example, studies have shown that acupuncture and acupressure can stimulate the release of endorphins, the body's natural painkillers, and reduce inflammation and oxidative stress. Other studies have shown that acupuncture and acupressure can modulate the autonomic nervous system, which controls many of the body's automatic functions, such as heart rate, blood pressure, and digestion.

Chi and Energy Flow

Chi is a fundamental concept in Traditional Chinese Medicine (TCM) and refers to the vital energy that animates all living beings and supports the body's functions. Chi is believed to flow through the meridian system, a network of energy channels that run throughout the body and are connected to the internal organs and physiological processes.

According to TCM, the balance and free flow of Chi are essential for maintaining health and preventing illness. When Chi is blocked or imbalanced, it can lead to various physical, emotional, and mental ailments.

The flow of Chi through the meridians can be stimulated through various techniques, such as acupuncture, acupressure, and Qi Gong. These techniques work by activating specific acupoints along the meridians, which can enhance the flow of Chi and promote healing and wellness.

The concept of Chi is also closely related to the concept of Yin and Yang, which are two opposing forces that are present in all things, including the body. In TCM, health is believed to be a state of balance between Yin and Yang, and imbalances between these forces can lead to various health conditions.

The flow of Chi is also connected to the body's circadian rhythm, with each meridian being most active during specific times of the day. For example, the Lung meridian is most active between 3-5am, while the Stomach meridian is most active between 7-9am.

While the concept of Chi is central to TCM, it has been the subject of much debate and skepticism in the West. However, modern research has shown that the meridian system and acupoints can be objectively measured and have distinct physiological and biochemical properties.

For example, studies have shown that acupuncture and acupressure can stimulate the release of endorphins, the body's natural painkillers, and reduce inflammation and oxidative stress. Other studies have shown that acupuncture and acupressure can modulate the autonomic nervous system, which controls many of the body's automatic functions, such as heart rate, blood pressure, and digestion.

Despite the skepticism and controversy surrounding the concept of Chi, many people have reported significant benefits from practicing techniques that stimulate the flow of Chi, such as Qi Gong and acupressure. These practices can help promote relaxation, reduce stress, and enhance overall well-being.

In addition to acupressure and Qi Gong, there are several other techniques that can be used to enhance the flow of Chi and promote healing and wellness. These include Tai Chi, yoga, meditation, and herbal remedies.

The Role of Pressure Points

Pressure points are specific areas on the body that can be stimulated to promote healing and wellness. In the context of acupressure, pressure points are acupoints located along the meridians, a network of energy channels that run throughout the body and are connected to the internal organs and physiological processes.

Each pressure point is associated with a specific meridian and organ system and can be stimulated to promote the flow of Qi, the vital energy that supports the body's functions. Pressure points can be stimulated through various techniques, such as acupressure, massage, and acupuncture.

Acupressure is a therapy that involves applying pressure on specific points on the body to stimulate the flow of Qi and promote healing. Acupressure can be performed with the fingers, thumbs, palms, or other tools, such as acupressure balls or mats.

One of the main benefits of acupressure is that it is non-invasive and can be performed by anyone with basic knowledge of the acupressure points and techniques. Acupressure can be used to complement conventional medical treatments and promote relaxation, reduce stress, and enhance overall well-being.

Acupuncture is another therapy that involves stimulating pressure points to promote healing and wellness. Unlike acupressure, acupuncture involves inserting thin needles into specific points on the body to stimulate the flow of Qi. Acupuncture is often combined with other therapies, such as cupping, moxibustion, or electrical stimulation, to enhance its effects.

The pressure points used in acupuncture and acupressure are based on the principles of Traditional Chinese Medicine (TCM), which views the body as a holistic system that is interconnected and interdependent. In TCM, health is believed to be a state of balance between Yin and Yang, two opposing forces that are present in all things, including the body.

When Qi is blocked or imbalanced, it can lead to various physical, emotional, and mental ailments. Stimulating pressure points can enhance the flow of Qi and promote balance and harmony within the body.

Pressure points can be used to treat a wide range of health conditions, from chronic pain and stress to anxiety and depression. For example, the "Gallbladder 20" point, located at the base of the skull, is often used to relieve headaches and neck pain, while the "Pericardium 6" point, located on the inner forearm, is often used to reduce nausea and anxiety.

It is important to note that pressure points should be stimulated with care and caution, as improper technique or overuse can lead to complications, such as bruising, soreness, or dizziness. It is also important to consult with a healthcare provider before starting any new therapy, especially if you have a medical condition or are taking any medications.

Chapter Three

Acupressure Techniques

Acupressure is a therapy that involves applying pressure to specific points on the body to stimulate the flow of vital energy, or Qi, and promote healing and wellness. Acupressure is a non-invasive and safe therapy that can be performed by anyone with basic knowledge of the acupressure points and techniques.

There are several acupressure techniques that can be used to stimulate pressure points and promote healing and wellness. Some of the most commonly used acupressure techniques include:

1. Finger pressure: This is the most basic and widely used acupressure technique. It involves applying pressure on specific points with the fingers, thumbs, or palms. The pressure is applied in a circular or back-and-forth motion for several seconds or minutes.

2. Knuckle pressure: This technique involves using the knuckles to apply pressure on specific points. The knuckles are used to apply deeper and more focused pressure than finger pressure. This technique is particularly effective for treating deep-seated pain and tension.

3. Palm pressure: This technique involves using the palm of the hand to apply pressure on larger areas of the body, such as the back, chest, or abdomen. The palm is used to apply broad and even pressure, which can help promote relaxation and release tension.

4. Acupressure tools: There are several tools that can be used to apply pressure on specific points, such as acupressure balls, mats, or rollers. These tools can be particularly effective for treating hard-to-reach areas, such as the back, neck, or feet.

5. Trigger point therapy: This technique involves applying pressure on specific points, called trigger points, which are areas of muscle tension and pain. Trigger point therapy can be particularly effective for treating chronic pain and muscle tension.

Acupressure can be used to treat a wide range of health conditions, from chronic pain and stress to anxiety and depression. Some of the most commonly treated conditions include:

6. Headaches and migraines: Acupressure can be used to relieve headaches and migraines by stimulating pressure points on the head and neck.

7. Back pain: Acupressure can be used to relieve back pain by stimulating pressure points on the back and along the spine.

8. Anxiety and depression: Acupressure can be used to reduce anxiety and depression by stimulating pressure points that promote relaxation and emotional balance.

9. Digestive issues: Acupressure can be used to relieve digestive issues, such as bloating, constipation, and indigestion, by stimulating pressure points on the abdomen and along the digestive tract.

10. Insomnia: Acupressure can be used to improve sleep quality and relieve insomnia by stimulating pressure points that promote relaxation and calmness.

It is important to note that acupressure should be used with care and caution, as improper technique or overuse can lead to complications, such as bruising, soreness, or dizziness. It is also important to consult with a healthcare provider before starting any new therapy, especially if you have a medical condition or are taking any medications.

The Proper Application of Pressure

Acupressure is a therapy that involves applying pressure to specific points on the body to stimulate the flow of vital energy, or Qi, and promote healing and wellness. The proper application of pressure is crucial for effective acupressure and to prevent injury or discomfort.

When applying pressure, it is important to start with light pressure and gradually increase the intensity to a comfortable level. Acupressure should never be painful or cause discomfort. If you experience pain or discomfort, reduce the pressure or stop the therapy.

The pressure should be applied in a circular or back-and-forth motion for several seconds or minutes, depending on the acupressure point and the condition being treated. The pressure should be firm and even, and applied with the fingertips, thumbs, palms, or other tools, such as acupressure balls or mats.

The proper application of pressure depends on several factors, including the acupressure point location, the level of sensitivity, and the underlying condition being treated. Some acupressure points, such as those on the hands and feet, are more sensitive than others and require less pressure.

It is also important to avoid applying pressure to certain areas of the body, such as the eyes, throat, or genitals, as this can cause injury or discomfort. It is also important to avoid applying pressure over broken skin, wounds, or infections, as this can increase the risk of infection or inflammation.

When performing acupressure on yourself or others, it is important to use proper body mechanics to avoid strain or injury. For example, if you are applying pressure to a point on the back, you should stand or sit in a comfortable and stable position and use your body weight to apply the pressure, rather than straining your arms or shoulders.

It is also important to use proper hygiene when performing acupressure. Your hands should be clean and free of any cuts or infections, and any tools used for acupressure should be sanitized before and after each use.

In addition to proper pressure application, there are several other factors that can affect the effectiveness of acupressure, such as timing, duration, and frequency. Some acupressure points are most effective when stimulated at specific times of the day or night, while others can be stimulated at any time.

The duration and frequency of acupressure therapy depend on the condition being treated and the individual's response to therapy. For acute conditions, such as headaches or muscle tension, acupressure can be performed for several minutes, several times a day. For chronic conditions, such as anxiety or depression, acupressure may need to be performed regularly over several weeks or months to achieve the desired results.

Reflexology and Zone Therapy

Reflexology and Zone Therapy are two techniques that are closely related to acupressure, and involve the application of pressure to specific points on the body to promote healing and wellness. While acupressure is based on Traditional Chinese Medicine, Reflexology and Zone Therapy are based on different theories and approaches.

Reflexology is a therapy that involves the application of pressure to specific points on the feet, hands, and ears, known as reflex points, to stimulate the corresponding organs and systems in the body. Reflexology is based on the theory that the feet, hands, and ears contain reflex points that correspond to different parts of the body, and that by stimulating these points, the body's natural healing processes can be activated.

Reflexology is often used to promote relaxation, reduce stress, and improve circulation. It can also be used to treat a wide range of health conditions, including chronic pain, digestive issues, hormonal imbalances, and respiratory problems.

Zone Therapy is a therapy that involves the application of pressure to specific zones on the feet, hands, and ears, to promote healing and wellness. Zone Therapy is based on the theory that the body is divided into ten zones, each of which corresponds to different organs and systems in the body.

Zone Therapy is often used to promote relaxation, reduce stress, and improve circulation. It can also be used to treat a wide range of health conditions, including chronic pain, digestive issues, hormonal imbalances, and respiratory problems.

While Reflexology and Zone Therapy are different techniques, they both involve the application of pressure to specific points or zones on the body to promote healing and wellness. Both techniques are safe and non-invasive, and can be performed by anyone with proper training and knowledge.

In addition to the application of pressure, Reflexology and Zone Therapy also involve the use of massage and other techniques to enhance the effects of therapy. For example, Reflexology often involves the use of massage, stretching, and other techniques to relax and loosen the feet and hands, and to enhance the flow of Qi and blood in the body.

Zone Therapy often involves the use of acupressure, massage, and other techniques to stimulate the flow of Qi and promote balance and harmony within the body. Zone Therapy can be particularly effective for treating chronic pain and tension, as it targets specific zones and areas of the body that are often affected by these conditions.

Chapter Four

The Five Elements Theory

The Five Elements Theory is an important concept in Traditional Chinese Medicine and is closely related to the practice of acupressure. The Five Elements Theory is based on the idea that there are five elements, or phases, that represent different aspects of nature, including wood, fire, earth, metal, and water. Each element is associated with specific organs, emotions, colors, and seasons, and plays a crucial role in maintaining balance and harmony within the body.

The Five Elements Theory is used to understand the relationships between different organs and systems in the body, and to diagnose and treat a wide range of health conditions. The theory is also used to understand the emotional and spiritual aspects of health and wellness, and to promote overall well-being.

The wood element is associated with the liver and gallbladder organs, and is associated with growth, flexibility, and creativity. The wood element is also associated with the color green, the emotion of anger, and the season of spring. When the wood element is imbalanced, it can lead to issues such as depression, anxiety, and irritability.

The fire element is associated with the heart and small intestine organs, and is associated with passion, joy, and intimacy. The fire element is also associated with the color red, the emotion of happiness, and the season of summer. When the fire element is imbalanced, it can lead to issues such as insomnia, palpitations, and restlessness.

The earth element is associated with the spleen and stomach organs, and is associated with nourishment, grounding, and stability. The earth element is also associated with the color yellow, the emotion of worry, and the season of late summer. When the earth element is imbalanced, it can lead to issues such as digestive problems, fatigue, and overthinking.

The metal element is associated with the lung and large intestine organs, and is associated with inspiration, courage, and release. The metal element is also associated with the color white, the emotion of grief, and the season of autumn. When the metal element is imbalanced, it can lead to issues such as respiratory problems, skin disorders, and sadness.

The water element is associated with the kidney and bladder organs, and is associated with reflection, courage, and flow. The water element is also associated with the color black, the emotion of fear, and the season of winter. When the water element is imbalanced, it can lead to issues such as urinary problems, lower back pain, and lack of motivation.

Acupressure is used to stimulate specific points on the body that correspond to different organs and systems in the body, and can be used to balance the different elements and promote overall well-being. For example, acupressure points on the liver meridian can be used to treat imbalances in the wood element, while acupressure points on the kidney meridian can be used to treat imbalances in the water element.

In addition to acupressure, the Five Elements Theory is used in other forms of Traditional Chinese Medicine, such as acupuncture, herbal medicine, and Qigong. The theory is also used in other forms of holistic healing, such as yoga, meditation, and Ayurveda.

Common Acupressure Points

Acupressure is a therapy that involves the application of pressure to specific points on the body to stimulate the flow of vital energy, or Qi, and promote healing and wellness. There are many acupressure points on the body, each of which is associated with different organs, systems, and functions. Here are some common acupressure points and their uses:

1. LI4: Located between the thumb and index finger, LI4 is commonly used to relieve headaches, sinus pain, and toothaches. It is also used to promote labor during childbirth.

2. LV3: Located on the top of the foot, between the big toe and second toe, LV3 is commonly used to relieve stress, anxiety, and depression. It is also used to treat menstrual cramps and digestive problems.

3. ST36: Located on the lower leg, about four finger widths below the kneecap, ST36 is commonly used to relieve fatigue, boost immunity, and improve digestion. It is also used to treat menstrual cramps and respiratory problems.

4. PC6: Located on the inner forearm, about two finger widths from the wrist crease, PC6 is commonly used to relieve nausea, vomiting, and motion sickness. It is also used to treat anxiety and insomnia.

5. GB20: Located on the back of the head, in the hollows on either side of the neck, GB20 is commonly used to relieve headaches, neck pain, and eye strain. It is also used to treat insomnia and anxiety.

6. CV17: Located in the center of the chest, between the nipples, CV17 is commonly used to relieve stress, anxiety, and depression. It is also used to treat respiratory problems and promote overall well-being.

7. BL60: Located on the ankle, behind the ankle bone, BL60 is commonly used to relieve lower back pain, hip pain, and sciatica. It is also used to treat insomnia and anxiety.

8. GV20: Located on the top of the head, in the center of the scalp, GV20 is commonly used to relieve stress, anxiety, and depression. It is also used to treat migraines and promote overall well-being.

9. K1: Located on the sole of the foot, at the center of the heel, K1 is commonly used to relieve fatigue, improve circulation, and promote overall well-being. It is also used to treat insomnia and anxiety.

10. LI11: Located on the outer elbow, in the crease of the arm, LI11 is commonly used to relieve pain, inflammation, and fever. It is also used to treat digestive problems and promote overall well-being.

When applying pressure to these acupressure points, it is important to use proper technique and avoid causing pain or discomfort. The pressure should be applied in a circular or back-and-forth motion for several seconds or minutes, depending on the acupressure point and the condition being treated. It is also important to use proper hygiene and body mechanics to avoid injury or strain.

Acupressure is a safe and effective therapy that can be used to promote healing and wellness when performed with proper technique and care. If you are considering using acupressure for a specific condition, it is important to consult with a qualified healthcare practitioner to determine the best approach for your individual needs.

Points for Pain Relief

Acupressure is a therapy that has been used for centuries to treat pain and promote healing. There are many acupressure points on the body that can be used to relieve pain and discomfort, including headaches, back pain, and menstrual cramps. Here are some common acupressure points for pain relief:

1. GB20: Located on the back of the head, in the hollows on either side of the neck, GB20 is commonly used to relieve headaches and migraines. Applying pressure to GB20 can help to relax the neck muscles and promote blood flow to the head, which can reduce the intensity and frequency of headaches.

2. LI4: Located between the thumb and index finger, LI4 is commonly used to relieve headaches, toothaches, and sinus pain. Applying pressure to LI4 can help to stimulate the flow of Qi and blood in the body, which can reduce pain and inflammation.

3. ST36: Located on the lower leg, about four finger widths below the kneecap, ST36 is commonly used to relieve lower back pain, knee pain, and menstrual cramps. Applying pressure to ST36 can help to improve circulation and reduce inflammation in the affected area.

4. BL60: Located on the ankle, behind the ankle bone, BL60 is commonly used to relieve lower back pain, hip pain, and sciatica. Applying pressure to BL60 can help to release tension in the muscles and promote blood flow to the affected area, which can reduce pain and improve mobility.

5. PC6: Located on the inner forearm, about two finger widths from the wrist crease, PC6 is commonly used to relieve nausea, vomiting, and motion sickness. Applying pressure to PC6 can help to stimulate the flow of Qi and blood in the body, which can reduce feelings of nausea and promote relaxation.

6. K1: Located on the sole of the foot, at the center of the heel, K1 is commonly used to relieve fatigue, improve circulation, and promote overall well-being. Applying pressure to K1 can help to stimulate the flow of Qi and blood in the body, which can reduce pain and promote relaxation.

7. CV12: Located on the front of the body, in the center of the chest, CV12 is commonly used to relieve stomach pain, indigestion, and acid reflux. Applying pressure to CV12 can help to improve digestion and reduce inflammation in the stomach and digestive tract.

8. GV20: Located on the top of the head, in the center of the scalp, GV20 is commonly used to relieve stress, anxiety, and depression. Applying pressure to GV20 can help to promote relaxation and reduce feelings of tension and anxiety.

9. LI11: Located on the outer elbow, in the crease of the arm, LI11 is commonly used to relieve pain, inflammation, and fever. Applying pressure to LI11 can help to stimulate the immune system and promote healing.

10. LV3: Located on the top of the foot, between the big toe and second toe, LV3 is commonly used to relieve stress, anxiety, and menstrual cramps. Applying pressure to LV3 can help to stimulate the flow of Qi and blood in the body, which can reduce pain and promote relaxation.

Acupressure is a safe and effective therapy that can be used to relieve pain and promote healing when performed with proper technique and care. If you are considering using acupressure for pain relief, it is important to consult with a qualified healthcare practitioner to determine the best approach for your individual needs. With the right approach, acupressure can be an effective tool for managing pain and promoting overall well-being.

Points for Stress Reduction

Stress is a common problem that can have a significant impact on physical, emotional, and mental health. Acupressure is a therapy that has been used for centuries to promote relaxation and reduce stress. There are many acupressure points on the body that can be used to promote relaxation and reduce feelings of tension and anxiety. Here are some common acupressure points for stress reduction:

1. GV20: Located on the top of the head, in the center of the scalp, GV20 is commonly used to relieve stress, anxiety, and depression. Applying pressure to GV20 can help to promote relaxation and reduce feelings of tension and anxiety.

2. LI4: Located between the thumb and index finger, LI4 is commonly used to relieve stress, anxiety, and tension. Applying pressure to LI4 can help to stimulate the flow of Qi and blood in the body, which can promote relaxation and reduce feelings of anxiety and tension.

3. PC6: Located on the inner forearm, about two finger widths from the wrist crease, PC6 is commonly used to relieve stress, anxiety, and nausea. Applying pressure to PC6 can help to promote relaxation and reduce feelings of tension and anxiety, as well as reduce feelings of nausea and promote overall well-being.

4. CV17: Located in the center of the chest, between the nipples, CV17 is commonly used to relieve stress, anxiety, and depression. Applying pressure to CV17 can help to promote relaxation and reduce feelings of tension and anxiety, as well as improve respiratory function and promote overall well-being.

5. LV3: Located on the top of the foot, between the big toe and second toe, LV3 is commonly used to relieve stress, anxiety, and promote relaxation. Applying pressure to LV3 can help to stimulate the flow of Qi and blood in the body, which can promote relaxation and reduce feelings of tension and anxiety.

6. BL10: Located at the base of the skull, in the hollows on either side of the neck, BL10 is commonly used to relieve stress, anxiety, and tension

headaches. Applying pressure to BL10 can help to promote relaxation and reduce feelings of tension and anxiety, as well as reduce the intensity and frequency of tension headaches.

7. ST36: Located on the lower leg, about four finger widths below the kneecap, ST36 is commonly used to relieve stress, anxiety, and fatigue. Applying pressure to ST36 can help to promote relaxation and reduce feelings of tension and anxiety, as well as improve energy levels and promote overall well-being.

8. K1: Located on the sole of the foot, at the center of the heel, K1 is commonly used to relieve stress, anxiety, and promote relaxation. Applying pressure to K1 can help to stimulate the flow of Qi and blood in the body, which can promote relaxation and reduce feelings of tension and anxiety.

9. GB20: Located on the back of the head, in the hollows on either side of the neck, GB20 is commonly used to relieve stress, anxiety, and tension headaches. Applying pressure to GB20 can help to promote relaxation and reduce feelings of tension and anxiety, as well as reduce the intensity and frequency of tension headaches.

10. Yintang: Located between the eyebrows, at the center of the forehead, Yintang is commonly used to relieve stress, anxiety, and promote relaxation. Applying pressure to Yintang can help to promote relaxation and reduce feelings of tension and anxiety, as well as promote mental clarity and focus.

Acupressure is a safe and effective therapy that can be used to promote relaxation and reduce stress when performed with proper technique and care. If you are considering using acupressure for stress reduction, it is important to consult with a qualified healthcare practitioner to

Points for Digestive Health

Digestive health is essential for overall well-being, but many people struggle with digestive issues such as indigestion, bloating, and constipation. Acupressure is a therapy that has been used for centuries to promote digestive health and relieve digestive issues. There are many acupressure points on the body that can be used to promote digestion and relieve digestive issues. Here are some common acupressure points for digestive health:

1. CV12: Located on the front of the body, in the center of the chest, CV12 is commonly used to relieve digestive issues such as indigestion, bloating, and acid reflux. Applying pressure to CV12 can help to improve digestion and reduce inflammation in the stomach and digestive tract.

2. ST36: Located on the lower leg, about four finger widths below the kneecap, ST36 is commonly used to promote digestion and relieve digestive issues such as bloating, constipation, and diarrhea. Applying pressure to ST36 can help to improve circulation and reduce inflammation in the digestive tract.

3. PC6: Located on the inner forearm, about two finger widths from the wrist crease, PC6 is commonly used to relieve nausea and promote digestion. Applying pressure to PC6 can help to stimulate the flow of Qi and blood in the body, which can reduce feelings of nausea and promote overall digestive health.

4. SP6: Located on the inner leg, about four finger widths above the ankle bone, SP6 is commonly used to promote digestion and relieve digestive issues such as bloating and constipation. Applying pressure to SP6 can help to improve circulation and reduce inflammation in the digestive tract.

5. LI4: Located between the thumb and index finger, LI4 is commonly used to relieve digestive issues such as constipation and diarrhea. Applying

pressure to LI4 can help to stimulate the flow of Qi and blood in the body, which can promote digestion and relieve digestive issues.

6. BL21: Located on the lower back, on either side of the spine, BL21 is commonly used to promote digestion and relieve digestive issues such as constipation and diarrhea. Applying pressure to BL21 can help to improve circulation and reduce inflammation in the digestive tract.

7. CV6: Located on the lower abdomen, about two finger widths below the belly button, CV6 is commonly used to promote digestion and relieve digestive issues such as bloating and constipation. Applying pressure to CV6 can help to stimulate the flow of Qi and blood in the body, which can improve digestion and relieve digestive issues.

8. LR3: Located on the top of the foot, between the big toe and second toe, LR3 is commonly used to promote digestion and relieve digestive issues such as constipation and diarrhea. Applying pressure to LR3 can help to stimulate the flow of Qi and blood in the body, which can improve digestion and relieve digestive issues.

9. GB34: Located on the outer leg, below the knee, GB34 is commonly used to promote digestion and relieve digestive issues such as bloating and constipation. Applying pressure to GB34 can help to improve circulation and reduce inflammation in the digestive tract.

10. K27: Located on the chest, on either side of the sternum, K27 is commonly used to promote digestion and relieve digestive issues such as acid reflux and indigestion. Applying pressure to K27 can help to improve respiratory function and reduce inflammation in the digestive tract.

Acupressure is a safe and effective therapy that can be used to promote digestive health and relieve digestive issues when performed with proper technique and care. If you are considering using acupressure for digestive health, it is important to consult with a qualified healthcare practitioner to determine the best approach for your individual needs. With the right approach, acupressure can be

Chapter Five

Acupressure for Emotional Well-being

Emotional well-being is essential for overall health and happiness, but many people struggle with emotional issues such as anxiety, depression, and stress. Acupressure is a therapy that has been used for centuries to promote emotional well-being and relieve emotional issues. There are many acupressure points on the body that can be used to promote emotional balance and relieve emotional issues. Here are some common acupressure points for emotional well-being:

1. Yintang: Located between the eyebrows, at the center of the forehead, Yintang is commonly used to relieve anxiety, stress, and promote relaxation. Applying pressure to Yintang can help to promote mental clarity and focus, as well as reduce feelings of anxiety and stress.

2. CV17: Located in the center of the chest, between the nipples, CV17 is commonly used to relieve stress, anxiety, and depression. Applying pressure to CV17 can help to promote relaxation and reduce feelings of tension and anxiety, as well as improve respiratory function and promote overall well-being.

3. LI4: Located between the thumb and index finger, LI4 is commonly used to relieve stress, anxiety, and tension. Applying pressure to LI4 can help to stimulate the flow of Qi and blood in the body, which can promote relaxation and reduce feelings of anxiety and tension.

4. PC6: Located on the inner forearm, about two finger widths from the wrist crease, PC6 is commonly used to relieve anxiety, stress, and nausea. Applying pressure to PC6 can help to promote relaxation and reduce feelings of tension and anxiety, as well as reduce feelings of nausea and promote overall well-being.

5. GB20: Located on the back of the head, in the hollows on either side of the neck, GB20 is commonly used to relieve stress, anxiety, and tension headaches. Applying pressure to GB20 can help to promote relaxation and reduce feelings of tension and anxiety, as well as reduce the intensity and frequency of tension headaches.

6. BL10: Located at the base of the skull, in the hollows on either side of the neck, BL10 is commonly used to relieve stress, anxiety, and tension headaches. Applying pressure to BL10 can help to promote relaxation and reduce feelings of tension and anxiety, as well as reduce the intensity and frequency of tension headaches.

7. GV20: Located on the top of the head, in the center of the scalp, GV20 is commonly used to relieve stress, anxiety, and depression. Applying pressure to GV20 can help to promote relaxation and reduce feelings of tension and anxiety.

8. HT7: Located on the inner wrist, at the crease of the wrist, HT7 is commonly used to relieve anxiety, depression, and promote relaxation. Applying pressure to HT7 can help to stimulate the flow of Qi and blood in the body, which can reduce feelings of anxiety and depression and promote overall emotional well-being.

9. SP6: Located on the inner leg, about four finger widths above the ankle bone, SP6 is commonly used to relieve anxiety, stress, and promote relaxation. Applying pressure to SP6 can help to improve circulation and reduce feelings of tension and anxiety.

10. LR3: Located on the top of the foot, between the big toe and second toe, LR3 is commonly used to relieve stress, anxiety, and promote relaxation. Applying pressure to LR3 can help to stimulate the flow of Qi and blood in the body, which can promote relaxation and reduce feelings of tension and anxiety.

Acupressure is a safe and effective therapy that can be used to promote emotional well-being and relieve emotional issues when performed with proper technique and care. If you are considering using acupressure for emotional well-being, it is important to consult with a qualified healthcare practitioner to

Balancing Emotions

Emotional balance is essential for overall well-being, but many people struggle with emotional imbalances such as anxiety, depression, and mood swings. Acupressure is a therapy that has been used for centuries to promote emotional balance and relieve emotional imbalances. There are many acupressure points on the body that can be used to promote emotional balance and relieve emotional imbalances. Here are some common acupressure points for balancing emotions:

1. GV20: Located on the top of the head, in the center of the scalp, GV20 is commonly used to promote emotional balance and relieve emotional imbalances. Applying pressure to GV20 can help to stimulate the flow of Qi and blood in the body, which can promote emotional balance and reduce feelings of anxiety and depression.

2. CV17: Located in the center of the chest, between the nipples, CV17 is commonly used to promote emotional balance and relieve emotional imbalances such as anxiety and depression. Applying pressure to CV17 can

help to promote relaxation and reduce feelings of tension and anxiety, as well as improve respiratory function and promote overall well-being.

3. PC6: Located on the inner forearm, about two finger widths from the wrist crease, PC6 is commonly used to promote emotional balance and relieve emotional imbalances such as anxiety, stress, and nausea. Applying pressure to PC6 can help to promote relaxation and reduce feelings of tension and anxiety, as well as reduce feelings of nausea and promote overall well-being.

4. BL15: Located on the upper back, on either side of the spine, BL15 is commonly used to promote emotional balance and relieve emotional imbalances such as anxiety and depression. Applying pressure to BL15 can help to stimulate the flow of Qi and blood in the body, which can promote emotional balance and reduce feelings of anxiety and depression.

5. LI4: Located between the thumb and index finger, LI4 is commonly used to promote emotional balance and relieve emotional imbalances such as anxiety and tension. Applying pressure to LI4 can help to stimulate the flow of Qi and blood in the body, which can promote emotional balance and reduce feelings of anxiety and tension.

6. SP6: Located on the inner leg, about four finger widths above the ankle bone, SP6 is commonly used to promote emotional balance and relieve emotional imbalances such as anxiety and stress. Applying pressure to SP6 can help to improve circulation and reduce feelings of tension and anxiety.

7. HT7: Located on the inner wrist, at the crease of the wrist, HT7 is commonly used to promote emotional balance and relieve emotional imbalances such as anxiety and depression. Applying pressure to HT7 can help to stimulate the flow of Qi and blood in the body, which can reduce feelings of anxiety and depression and promote overall emotional well-being.

8. K27: Located on the chest, on either side of the sternum, K27 is commonly used to promote emotional balance and relieve emotional imbalances such as anxiety and depression. Applying pressure to K27 can help to improve respiratory function and promote emotional balance and well-being.

9. LR3: Located on the top of the foot, between the big toe and second toe, LR3 is commonly used to promote emotional balance and relieve emotional imbalances such as anxiety and stress. Applying pressure to LR3 can help to stimulate the flow of Qi and blood in the body, which can promote emotional balance and reduce feelings of anxiety and stress.

10. Yintang: Located between the eyebrows, at the center of the forehead, Yintang is commonly used to promote emotional balance and relieve emotional imbalances such as anxiety and stress. Applying pressure to Yintang can help to promote relaxation and reduce feelings of tension and anxiety.

Acupressure is a safe and effective therapy that can be used to

Overcoming Anxiety and Depression

Anxiety and depression are two common mental health issues that can affect anyone, regardless of age or gender. While there are many treatments available for anxiety and depression, acupressure is a safe and effective therapy that can be used to overcome these conditions. In this article, we will explore how acupressure can be used to overcome anxiety and depression.

What is Acupressure?

Acupressure is a therapy that has been used for centuries in Traditional Chinese Medicine to promote healing and wellness. The therapy involves applying pressure to specific points on the body, known as acupressure points, to stimulate the flow of energy, or Qi, throughout the body. By stimulating these points, acupressure can help to alleviate pain, reduce stress and anxiety, and improve overall well-being.

Acupressure Points for Anxiety and Depression

There are several acupressure points that can be used to overcome anxiety and depression. Here are some of the most commonly used points:

1. GV20: Located on the top of the head, in the center of the scalp, GV20 is commonly used to promote emotional balance and relieve emotional imbalances such as anxiety and depression. Applying pressure to GV20 can help to stimulate the flow of Qi and blood in the body, which can promote emotional balance and reduce feelings of anxiety and depression.

2. CV17: Located in the center of the chest, between the nipples, CV17 is commonly used to promote emotional balance and relieve emotional imbalances such as anxiety and depression. Applying pressure to CV17 can help to promote relaxation and reduce feelings of tension and anxiety, as well as improve respiratory function and promote overall well-being.

3. PC6: Located on the inner forearm, about two finger widths from the wrist crease, PC6 is commonly used to relieve anxiety, stress, and nausea. Applying pressure to PC6 can help to promote relaxation and reduce feelings of tension and anxiety, as well as reduce feelings of nausea and promote overall well-being.

4. BL15: Located on the upper back, on either side of the spine, BL15 is commonly used to promote emotional balance and relieve emotional imbalances such as anxiety and depression. Applying pressure to BL15 can help to stimulate the flow of Qi and blood in the body, which can promote emotional balance and reduce feelings of anxiety and depression.

5. LI4: Located between the thumb and index finger, LI4 is commonly used to promote emotional balance and relieve emotional imbalances such as anxiety and tension. Applying pressure to LI4 can help to stimulate the flow of Qi and blood in the body, which can promote emotional balance and reduce feelings of anxiety and tension.

Acupressure Techniques for Anxiety and Depression

There are several acupressure techniques that can be used to overcome anxiety and depression. Here are some of the most effective techniques:

6. Finger Pressure: Apply gentle pressure to the acupressure points using the fingers. Apply pressure for 30 seconds to 1 minute, and repeat the process several times a day.

7. Massage: Massage the acupressure points in a circular motion using the fingers. Massage for 1-2 minutes, and repeat the process several times a day.

8. Acupressure Mats: Acupressure mats are designed to stimulate the acupressure points on the body. Lay on the acupressure mat for 20-30 minutes a day to relieve stress and anxiety.

9. Acupressure Pens: Acupressure pens are designed to apply pressure to the acupressure points using a small metal ball. Apply pressure to the acupressure points using the acupressure pen for several minutes a day to relieve anxiety and depression.

Benefits of Acupressure for Anxiety

Enhancing Mental Clarity

In today's fast-paced world, mental clarity is essential for productivity and well-being. Acupressure is a therapy that can be used to enhance mental clarity and improve cognitive function. In this article, we will explore how acupressure can be used to enhance mental clarity.

What is Acupressure?

Acupressure is a therapy that involves applying pressure to specific points on the body to stimulate the flow of energy, or Qi, throughout the body. By stimulating these points, acupressure can help to alleviate pain, reduce stress and anxiety, and improve overall well-being.

Acupressure Points for Mental Clarity

There are several acupressure points that can be used to enhance mental clarity. Here are some of the most commonly used points:

1. GV20: Located on the top of the head, in the center of the scalp, GV20 is commonly used to promote mental clarity and relieve mental fatigue. Applying pressure to GV20 can help to stimulate the flow of Qi and blood in the body, which can improve cognitive function and promote mental clarity.

2. CV17: Located in the center of the chest, between the nipples, CV17 is commonly used to promote mental clarity and relieve mental fatigue. Applying pressure to CV17 can help to promote relaxation and reduce feelings of mental exhaustion, as well as improve respiratory function and promote overall well-being.

3. PC6: Located on the inner forearm, about two finger widths from the wrist crease, PC6 is commonly used to promote mental clarity and relieve mental fatigue. Applying pressure to PC6 can help to promote relaxation and reduce feelings of mental exhaustion, as well as promote overall well-being.

4. BL10: Located on the nape of the neck, BL10 is commonly used to promote mental clarity and relieve mental fatigue. Applying pressure to BL10 can help to stimulate the flow of Qi and blood in the body, which can improve cognitive function and promote mental clarity.

5. LI4: Located between the thumb and index finger, LI4 is commonly used to promote mental clarity and relieve mental fatigue. Applying pressure to LI4 can help to stimulate the flow of Qi and blood in the body, which can improve cognitive function and promote mental clarity.

Acupressure Techniques for Mental Clarity

There are several acupressure techniques that can be used to enhance mental clarity. Here are some of the most effective techniques:

6. Finger Pressure: Apply gentle pressure to the acupressure points using the fingers. Apply pressure for 30 seconds to 1 minute, and repeat the process several times a day.

7. Massage: Massage the acupressure points in a circular motion using the fingers. Massage for 1-2 minutes, and repeat the process several times a day.

8. Acupressure Mats: Acupressure mats are designed to stimulate the acupressure points on the body. Lay on the acupressure mat for 20-30 minutes a day to promote mental clarity and relieve mental fatigue.

9. Acupressure Pens: Acupressure pens are designed to apply pressure to the acupressure points using a small metal ball. Apply pressure to the acupressure points using the acupressure pen for several minutes a day to promote mental clarity and relieve mental fatigue.

Benefits of Acupressure for Mental Clarity

Acupressure can be a valuable tool for enhancing mental clarity and improving cognitive function. By stimulating the flow of Qi and blood in the body, acupressure can help to improve cognitive function and promote mental clarity. Acupressure can also help to relieve mental fatigue, reduce stress and anxiety, and promote overall well-being.

Chapter Six

Acupressure for Physical Health

Acupressure is an ancient therapy that has been used for thousands of years to promote physical health and well-being. The therapy involves applying pressure to specific points on the body to stimulate the flow of energy, or Qi, throughout the body. By stimulating these points, acupressure can help to alleviate pain, reduce inflammation, improve circulation, and promote overall physical health. In this article, we will explore how acupressure can be used to promote physical health.

What is Acupressure?

Acupressure is a therapy that involves applying pressure to specific points on the body to stimulate the flow of energy, or Qi, throughout the body. By stimulating these points, acupressure can help to alleviate pain, reduce inflammation, improve circulation, and promote overall physical health.

Acupressure Points for Physical Health

There are several acupressure points that can be used to promote physical health. Here are some of the most commonly used points:

1. LI4: Located between the thumb and index finger, LI4 is commonly used to relieve pain and promote physical well-being. Applying pressure to LI4 can help to stimulate the flow of Qi and blood in the body, which can help to reduce pain and promote overall physical health.

2. ST36: Located on the lower leg, about four finger widths below the kneecap, ST36 is commonly used to promote digestive health, reduce inflammation, and boost the immune system. Applying pressure to ST36 can help to improve digestion, reduce inflammation, and promote overall physical health.

3. GB34: Located on the outside of the lower leg, below the knee, GB34 is commonly used to relieve pain and promote overall physical health. Applying pressure to GB34 can help to stimulate the flow of Qi and blood in the body, which can help to reduce pain and promote overall physical health.

4. SP6: Located on the inner leg, about four finger widths above the ankle, SP6 is commonly used to promote reproductive health, relieve pain, and reduce inflammation. Applying pressure to SP6 can help to improve reproductive health, reduce pain, and promote overall physical health.

5. BL60: Located on the ankle, on the outside of the foot, BL60 is commonly used to relieve pain and promote overall physical health. Applying pressure to BL60 can help to stimulate the flow of Qi and blood in the body, which can help to reduce pain and promote overall physical health.

Acupressure Techniques for Physical Health

There are several acupressure techniques that can be used to promote physical health. Here are some of the most effective techniques:

6. Finger Pressure: Apply gentle pressure to the acupressure points using the fingers. Apply pressure for 30 seconds to 1 minute, and repeat the process several times a day.

7. Massage: Massage the acupressure points in a circular motion using the fingers. Massage for 1-2 minutes, and repeat the process several times a day.

8. Acupressure Mats: Acupressure mats are designed to stimulate the acupressure points on the body. Lay on the acupressure mat for 20-30 minutes a day to promote physical health and relieve pain.

9. Acupressure Pens: Acupressure pens are designed to apply pressure to the acupressure points using a small metal ball. Apply pressure to the acupressure points using the acupressure pen for several minutes a day to promote physical health and relieve pain.

Benefits of Acupressure for Physical Health

Acupressure can be a valuable tool for promoting physical health and well-being. By stimulating the flow of Qi and blood in the body, acupressure can help to reduce pain,

Boosting Immunity

A strong immune system is essential for good health and well-being. The immune system helps to protect the body against viruses, bacteria, and other harmful substances. Acupressure is a natural therapy that can help to boost the immune system and improve overall health. In this article, we will explore how acupressure can be used to boost immunity.

What is Acupressure?

Acupressure is a therapy that involves applying pressure to specific points on the body to stimulate the flow of energy, or Qi, throughout the body. By stimulating these points, acupressure can help to alleviate pain, reduce inflammation, improve circulation, and promote overall physical and mental health.

Acupressure Points for Boosting Immunity

There are several acupressure points that can be used to boost the immune system. Here are some of the most commonly used points:

1. LI4: Located between the thumb and index finger, LI4 is commonly used to boost the immune system and promote overall health. Applying pressure to LI4 can help to stimulate the flow of Qi and blood in the body, which can help to improve immune function and promote overall well-being.

2. SP6: Located on the inner leg, about four finger widths above the ankle, SP6 is commonly used to boost the immune system and promote overall health. Applying pressure to SP6 can help to stimulate the flow of Qi and blood in the body, which can help to improve immune function and promote overall well-being.

3. GV14: Located on the upper back, in the center of the shoulder blades, GV14 is commonly used to boost the immune system and promote overall health. Applying pressure to GV14 can help to stimulate the flow of Qi and blood in the body, which can help to improve immune function and promote overall well-being.

4. BL11: Located on the back, on either side of the spine, BL11 is commonly used to boost the immune system and promote overall health. Applying pressure to BL11 can help to stimulate the flow of Qi and blood in the body, which can help to improve immune function and promote overall well-being.

5. CV6: Located on the lower abdomen, about two finger widths below the navel, CV6 is commonly used to boost the immune system and promote overall health. Applying pressure to CV6 can help to stimulate the flow of Qi and blood in the body, which can help to improve immune function and promote overall well-being.

Acupressure Techniques for Boosting Immunity

There are several acupressure techniques that can be used to boost the immune system. Here are some of the most effective techniques:

6. Finger Pressure: Apply gentle pressure to the acupressure points using the fingers. Apply pressure for 30 seconds to 1 minute, and repeat the process several times a day.

7. Massage: Massage the acupressure points in a circular motion using the fingers. Massage for 1-2 minutes, and repeat the process several times a day.

8. Acupressure Mats: Acupressure mats are designed to stimulate the acupressure points on the body. Lay on the acupressure mat for 20-30 minutes a day to promote immune function and improve overall health.

9. Acupressure Pens: Acupressure pens are designed to apply pressure to the acupressure points using a small metal ball. Apply pressure to the acupressure points using the acupressure pen for several minutes a day to boost immune function and improve overall health.

Benefits of Acupressure for Boosting Immunity

Acupressure can be a valuable tool for boosting the immune system and improving overall health. By stimulating the flow of Qi and blood in the

Improving Sleep Quality

A good night's sleep is essential for physical and mental well-being. However, many people struggle with sleep issues, such as insomnia or poor sleep quality. Acupressure is a natural therapy that can help to improve sleep quality and promote relaxation. In this article, we will explore how acupressure can be used to improve sleep quality.

What is Acupressure?

Acupressure is a therapy that involves applying pressure to specific points on the body to stimulate the flow of energy, or Qi, throughout the body. By stimulating these points, acupressure can help to alleviate pain, reduce inflammation, improve circulation, and promote overall physical and mental health.

Acupressure Points for Improving Sleep Quality

There are several acupressure points that can be used to improve sleep quality. Here are some of the most commonly used points:

1. HT7: Located on the wrist, on the pinky side, HT7 is commonly used to promote relaxation and improve sleep quality. Applying pressure to HT7 can help to calm the mind and promote deep, restful sleep.

2. GV20: Located on the top of the head, in the center, GV20 is commonly used to promote relaxation and improve sleep quality. Applying pressure to GV20 can help to calm the mind and promote deep, restful sleep.

3. PC6: Located on the inner arm, two finger widths above the wrist, PC6 is commonly used to promote relaxation and improve sleep quality. Applying pressure to PC6 can help to calm the mind and promote deep, restful sleep.

4. SP6: Located on the inner leg, about four finger widths above the ankle, SP6 is commonly used to promote relaxation and improve sleep quality. Applying pressure to SP6 can help to calm the mind and promote deep, restful sleep.

5. KI6: Located on the inner ankle, on the inside of the ankle bone, KI6 is commonly used to promote relaxation and improve sleep quality.

Applying pressure to KI6 can help to calm the mind and promote deep, restful sleep.

Acupressure Techniques for Improving Sleep Quality

There are several acupressure techniques that can be used to improve sleep quality. Here are some of the most effective techniques:

6. Finger Pressure: Apply gentle pressure to the acupressure points using the fingers. Apply pressure for 30 seconds to 1 minute, and repeat the process several times a day.

7. Massage: Massage the acupressure points in a circular motion using the fingers. Massage for 1-2 minutes, and repeat the process several times a day.

8. Acupressure Mats: Acupressure mats are designed to stimulate the acupressure points on the body. Lay on the acupressure mat for 20-30 minutes before bedtime to promote relaxation and improve sleep quality.

9. Acupressure Pens: Acupressure pens are designed to apply pressure to the acupressure points using a small metal ball. Apply pressure to the acupressure points using the acupressure pen for several minutes before bedtime to promote relaxation and improve sleep quality.

Benefits of Acupressure for Improving Sleep Quality

Acupressure can be a valuable tool for improving sleep quality and promoting relaxation. By stimulating the flow of Qi and blood in the body, acupressure can help to calm the mind, reduce stress and anxiety, and promote deep, restful sleep. Improved sleep quality can lead to better physical and mental health, increased energy levels, and a greater sense of well-being.

Increasing Energy Levels

In today's fast-paced world, many people struggle with low energy levels and fatigue. While there are many factors that can contribute to low energy levels, such as poor diet and lack of sleep, acupressure can be a natural and effective therapy for increasing energy levels. In this article, we will explore how acupressure can be used to increase energy levels.

What is Acupressure?

Acupressure is a therapy that involves applying pressure to specific points on the body to stimulate the flow of energy, or Qi, throughout the body. By stimulating these points, acupressure can help to alleviate pain, reduce inflammation, improve circulation, and promote overall physical and mental health.

Acupressure Points for Increasing Energy Levels

There are several acupressure points that can be used to increase energy levels. Here are some of the most commonly used points:

1. GV20: Located on the top of the head, in the center, GV20 is commonly used to increase energy levels and promote overall health. Applying pressure to GV20 can help to stimulate the flow of Qi and blood in the body, which can increase energy levels and promote overall well-being.

2. ST36: Located on the lower leg, about four finger widths below the kneecap, ST36 is commonly used to increase energy levels and promote overall health. Applying pressure to ST36 can help to stimulate the flow of Qi and blood in the body, which can increase energy levels and promote overall well-being.

3. CV6: Located on the lower abdomen, about two finger widths below the navel, CV6 is commonly used to increase energy levels and promote overall health. Applying pressure to CV6 can help to stimulate the flow of

Qi and blood in the body, which can increase energy levels and promote overall well-being.

4. BL23: Located on the lower back, on either side of the spine, BL23 is commonly used to increase energy levels and promote overall health. Applying pressure to BL23 can help to stimulate the flow of Qi and blood in the body, which can increase energy levels and promote overall well-being.

5. PC6: Located on the inner arm, two finger widths above the wrist, PC6 is commonly used to increase energy levels and promote overall health. Applying pressure to PC6 can help to stimulate the flow of Qi and blood in the body, which can increase energy levels and promote overall well-being.

Acupressure Techniques for Increasing Energy Levels

There are several acupressure techniques that can be used to increase energy levels. Here are some of the most effective techniques:

6. Finger Pressure: Apply gentle pressure to the acupressure points using the fingers. Apply pressure for 30 seconds to 1 minute, and repeat the process several times a day.

7. Massage: Massage the acupressure points in a circular motion using the fingers. Massage for 1-2 minutes, and repeat the process several times a day.

8. Acupressure Mats: Acupressure mats are designed to stimulate the acupressure points on the body. Lay on the acupressure mat for 20-30 minutes a day to increase energy levels and promote overall well-being.

9. Acupressure Pens: Acupressure pens are designed to apply pressure to the acupressure points using a small metal ball. Apply pressure to the acupressure points using the acupressure pen for several minutes a day to increase energy levels and promote overall well-being.

Benefits of Acupressure for Increasing Energy Levels

Acupressure can be a valuable tool for increasing energy levels and promoting overall well-being. By stimulating the flow of Qi and blood in the body, acupressure can help

Chapter Seven

Acupressure for Women's Health

Acupressure is an ancient healing technique that has been used for thousands of years to promote overall health and well-being. It involves applying pressure to specific points on the body to stimulate the flow of energy, or Qi, throughout the body. Acupressure can be a powerful tool for women's health, as it can help to alleviate menstrual pain, promote fertility, and ease the symptoms of menopause. In this article, we will explore how acupressure can be used for women's health.

Acupressure for Menstrual Pain

Many women experience menstrual pain and cramping during their menstrual cycle. Acupressure can be a natural and effective therapy for reducing menstrual pain and cramping. Here are some of the most commonly used acupressure points for menstrual pain:

1. SP6: Located on the inner leg, four finger widths above the ankle bone, SP6 is commonly used to relieve menstrual pain and cramping. Applying pressure to SP6 can help to stimulate the flow of Qi and blood in the body, which can reduce pain and promote overall well-being.

2. CV6: Located on the lower abdomen, about two finger widths below the navel, CV6 is commonly used to relieve menstrual pain and cramping. Applying pressure to CV6 can help to stimulate the flow of Qi and blood in the body, which can reduce pain and promote overall well-being.

3. LV3: Located on the top of the foot, between the big toe and second toe, LV3 is commonly used to relieve menstrual pain and cramping. Applying pressure to LV3 can help to stimulate the flow of Qi and blood in the body, which can reduce pain and promote overall well-being.

Acupressure for Fertility

Acupressure can also be used to promote fertility and increase the chances of conception. Here are some of the most commonly used acupressure points for fertility:

4. CV4: Located on the lower abdomen, about two finger widths below the navel, CV4 is commonly used to promote fertility. Applying pressure to CV4 can help to stimulate the reproductive organs and increase the chances of conception.

5. SP6: Located on the inner leg, four finger widths above the ankle bone, SP6 is commonly used to promote fertility. Applying pressure to SP6 can help to regulate the menstrual cycle and increase the chances of conception.

6. KI3: Located on the inner ankle, about one finger width behind the ankle bone, KI3 is commonly used to promote fertility. Applying pressure to KI3 can help to regulate the menstrual cycle and increase the chances of conception.

Acupressure for Menopause

Menopause can be a difficult time for many women, as it can be accompanied by a range of symptoms, including hot flashes, mood swings, and insomnia. Acupressure can be a natural and effective therapy for easing the symptoms of menopause. Here are some of the most commonly used acupressure points for menopause:

7. GV20: Located on the top of the head, in the center, GV20 is commonly used to ease the symptoms of menopause. Applying pressure to GV20 can help to regulate the hormonal balance in the body and reduce the frequency and intensity of hot flashes.

8. HT7: Located on the inner wrist, in the crease of the wrist, HT7 is commonly used to ease the symptoms of menopause. Applying pressure to HT7 can help to reduce anxiety and promote overall well-being.

9. SP6: Located on the inner leg, four finger widths above the ankle bone, SP6 is commonly used to ease the symptoms of menopause. Applying pressure to SP6 can help to regulate the menstrual cycle and reduce the frequency and intensity of hot

Menstrual Pain and Irregularities

Menstrual pain and irregularities are common issues that many women face. While medication and hormonal treatments are commonly used to manage these issues, there are also natural methods, such as acupressure, that can be used to alleviate menstrual pain and regulate the menstrual cycle. In this article, we will explore how acupressure can be used to address menstrual pain and irregularities.

Menstrual Pain

Menstrual pain, or dysmenorrhea, is a common issue that affects many women. The pain can range from mild to severe and can be accompanied by other symptoms such as cramping, bloating, and mood changes. Acupressure can be used as a natural and effective therapy for reducing menstrual pain. Here are some of the most commonly used acupressure points for menstrual pain:

1. SP6: Located on the inner leg, four finger widths above the ankle bone, SP6 is commonly used to relieve menstrual pain and cramping. Applying pressure to SP6 can help to stimulate the flow of Qi and blood in the body, which can reduce pain and promote overall well-being.

2. CV6: Located on the lower abdomen, about two finger widths below the navel, CV6 is commonly used to relieve menstrual pain and cramping. Applying pressure to CV6 can help to stimulate the flow of Qi and blood in the body, which can reduce pain and promote overall well-being.

3. LV3: Located on the top of the foot, between the big toe and second toe, LV3 is commonly used to relieve menstrual pain and cramping. Applying pressure to LV3 can help to stimulate the flow of Qi and blood in the body, which can reduce pain and promote overall well-being.

Menstrual Irregularities

Menstrual irregularities can include a range of issues, such as heavy bleeding, irregular cycles, and missed periods. Acupressure can be used to regulate the menstrual cycle and alleviate these issues. Here are some of the most commonly used acupressure points for menstrual irregularities:

4. CV4: Located on the lower abdomen, about two finger widths below the navel, CV4 is commonly used to regulate the menstrual cycle. Applying pressure to CV4 can help to stimulate the reproductive organs and regulate the menstrual cycle.

5. SP6: Located on the inner leg, four finger widths above the ankle bone, SP6 is commonly used to regulate the menstrual cycle. Applying pressure to SP6 can help to regulate the menstrual cycle and alleviate menstrual irregularities.

6. ST29: Located on the lower abdomen, about four finger widths below the navel, ST29 is commonly used to regulate the menstrual cycle. Apply-

ing pressure to ST29 can help to stimulate the reproductive organs and regulate the menstrual cycle.

Fertility and Pregnancy Support

Fertility and pregnancy support are important aspects of women's health, and acupressure can be a powerful tool for promoting reproductive health and supporting the journey to motherhood. In this article, we will explore how acupressure can be used to support fertility and pregnancy.

Fertility Support

Fertility issues are common among women, and can be caused by a range of factors including hormonal imbalances, stress, and reproductive disorders. Acupressure can be used to support fertility by regulating the menstrual cycle, reducing stress, and promoting reproductive health. Here are some of the most commonly used acupressure points for fertility support:

1. CV4: Located on the lower abdomen, about two finger widths below the navel, CV4 is commonly used to stimulate the reproductive organs and regulate the menstrual cycle. Applying pressure to CV4 can help to promote fertility by improving blood flow to the reproductive organs and regulating hormone levels.

2. SP6: Located on the inner leg, four finger widths above the ankle bone, SP6 is commonly used to stimulate the reproductive organs and regulate the menstrual cycle. Applying pressure to SP6 can help to promote fertility by improving blood flow to the reproductive organs and regulating hormone levels.

3. KD3: Located on the inner ankle, in the depression between the ankle bone and Achilles tendon, KD3 is commonly used to promote fertility

by improving kidney function. Applying pressure to KD3 can help to regulate the menstrual cycle and support overall reproductive health.

Pregnancy Support

Acupressure can also be used to support women during pregnancy, by reducing stress, alleviating common pregnancy symptoms, and promoting healthy labor and delivery. Here are some of the most commonly used acupressure points for pregnancy support:

4. PC6: Located on the inside of the wrist, about two finger widths from the crease of the wrist, PC6 is commonly used to alleviate nausea and morning sickness during pregnancy. Applying pressure to PC6 can help to reduce nausea and promote overall well-being during pregnancy.

5. BL32: Located in the lower back, at the level of the sacrum, BL32 is commonly used to relieve back pain during pregnancy. Applying pressure to BL32 can help to alleviate back pain and promote overall comfort during pregnancy.

6. LI4: Located on the webbing between the thumb and index finger, LI4 is commonly used to stimulate labor and promote healthy delivery. Applying pressure to LI4 can help to induce labor and reduce pain during delivery.

Menopause Relief

Menopause is a natural part of the aging process for women, but the symptoms that come with it can be challenging to manage. Hot flashes, mood swings, and insomnia are just a few of the common symptoms of menopause. While medication and hormone therapy are commonly used to manage these symptoms, acupressure can also be a natural and effective way to alleviate menopause symptoms. In this article, we will explore how acupressure can be used to provide relief during menopause.

Hot Flashes

Hot flashes are one of the most common symptoms of menopause, and can be both uncomfortable and disruptive to daily life. Acupressure can be used to alleviate hot flashes by promoting circulation and reducing stress. Here are some of the most commonly used acupressure points for hot flash relief:

1. HT7: Located on the inside of the wrist, HT7 is commonly used to alleviate hot flashes and reduce anxiety. Applying pressure to HT7 can help to promote circulation and reduce stress, which can alleviate hot flashes.

2. LI11: Located at the outer end of the elbow crease, LI11 is commonly used to alleviate hot flashes and promote overall well-being. Applying pressure to LI11 can help to regulate the flow of Qi and blood in the body, which can alleviate hot flashes.

3. GV20: Located at the top of the head, GV20 is commonly used to promote overall well-being and alleviate hot flashes. Applying pressure to GV20 can help to reduce stress and promote relaxation, which can alleviate hot flashes.

Mood Swings

Mood swings are another common symptom of menopause, and can be caused by fluctuating hormone levels. Acupressure can be used to alleviate mood swings by regulating hormone levels and promoting relaxation. Here are some of the most commonly used acupressure points for mood swing relief:

4. CV17: Located at the center of the chest, between the nipples, CV17 is commonly used to alleviate mood swings and promote relaxation. Applying pressure to CV17 can help to regulate hormone levels and promote emotional balance.

5. PC6: Located on the inside of the wrist, about two finger widths from the crease of the wrist, PC6 is commonly used to alleviate anxiety and promote emotional balance. Applying pressure to PC6 can help to promote relaxation and alleviate mood swings.

6. KD1: Located on the sole of the foot, at the depression when the foot is flexed, KD1 is commonly used to alleviate anxiety and promote relaxation. Applying pressure to KD1 can help to regulate hormone levels and promote emotional balance.

Insomnia

Insomnia is a common symptom of menopause, and can be caused by hormonal changes and hot flashes. Acupressure can be used to alleviate insomnia by promoting relaxation and reducing stress. Here are some of the most commonly used acupressure points for insomnia relief:

7. HT7: Located on the inside of the wrist, HT7 is commonly used to alleviate insomnia and promote relaxation. Applying pressure to HT7 can help to reduce stress and promote emotional balance, which can alleviate insomnia.

8. SP6: Located on the inner leg, four finger widths above the ankle bone, SP6 is commonly used to alleviate insomnia and promote relaxation. Applying pressure to SP6 can help to regulate hormone levels and promote emotional balance, which can alleviate insomnia.

9. GV20: Located at the top of the head, GV20 is commonly used to alleviate insomnia and promote relaxation. Applying pressure to GV20 can

help to reduce stress and promote emotional balance, which can alleviate insomnia.

Chapter Eight

Acupressure for Specific Conditions

Acupressure is a natural and effective way to manage a wide range of health conditions. By stimulating specific points on the body, acupressure can promote circulation, regulate hormone levels, reduce stress, and promote overall well-being. In this article, we will explore how acupressure can be used to manage specific health conditions.

Headaches

Headaches can be caused by a variety of factors, including stress, tension, and poor circulation. Acupressure can be used to manage headaches by promoting circulation and reducing stress. Here are some of the most commonly used acupressure points for headache relief:

1. LI4: Located in the fleshy webbing between the thumb and index finger, LI4 is commonly used to alleviate headaches and promote overall well-being. Applying pressure to LI4 can help to promote circulation and reduce stress, which can alleviate headaches.

2. GB20: Located at the base of the skull, in the hollows on either side of the neck, GB20 is commonly used to alleviate headaches and promote relaxation. Applying pressure to GB20 can help to promote circulation and reduce tension, which can alleviate headaches.

3. Yintang: Located between the eyebrows, Yintang is commonly used to alleviate headaches and promote relaxation. Applying pressure to Yintang

can help to reduce stress and promote emotional balance, which can alleviate headaches.

Allergies

Allergies are caused by an immune system response to a foreign substance, such as pollen or dust. Acupressure can be used to manage allergies by regulating the immune system and promoting overall well-being. Here are some of the most commonly used acupressure points for allergy relief:

4. LI11: Located at the outer end of the elbow crease, LI11 is commonly used to regulate the immune system and promote overall well-being. Applying pressure to LI11 can help to reduce inflammation and promote healing, which can alleviate allergies.

5. LU5: Located on the inside of the forearm, about two finger widths above the wrist, LU5 is commonly used to regulate the immune system and promote overall well-being. Applying pressure to LU5 can help to promote circulation and reduce inflammation, which can alleviate allergies.

6. GV14: Located at the base of the neck, between the shoulder blades, GV14 is commonly used to regulate the immune system and promote overall well-being. Applying pressure to GV14 can help to reduce stress and promote relaxation, which can alleviate allergies.

Back Pain

Back pain can be caused by a variety of factors, including poor posture, muscle strain, and injury. Acupressure can be used to manage back pain by promoting circulation and reducing tension. Here are some of the most commonly used acupressure points for back pain relief:

7. UB23: Located on the lower back, about two finger widths from the spine, UB23 is commonly used to alleviate back pain and promote overall

well-being. Applying pressure to UB23 can help to promote circulation and reduce tension, which can alleviate back pain.

8. GB30: Located in the buttocks, halfway between the hip joint and the base of the spine, GB30 is commonly used to alleviate back pain and promote relaxation. Applying pressure to GB30 can help to promote circulation and reduce tension, which can alleviate back pain.

9. BL60: Located on the foot, in the depression between the ankle bone and the Achilles tendon, BL60 is commonly used to alleviate back pain and promote overall well-being. Applying pressure to BL60 can help to promote circulation and reduce tension, which can alleviate back pain.

Digestive Issues

Digestive issues, such as indigestion and bloating, can be caused by a variety of factors, including poor diet, stress, and hormonal imbalances. Ac

Headaches and Migraines

Headaches and migraines are a common condition that can be debilitating and affect daily life. Traditional medicine treatments for headaches and migraines often include over-the-counter medications or prescription drugs. However, more and more people are turning to natural remedies like acupressure to alleviate their symptoms. In this article, we will explore how acupressure can be used to manage headaches and migraines.

What are headaches and migraines?

Headaches are a common condition that causes pain and discomfort in the head and neck area. There are several types of headaches, including tension headaches, cluster headaches, and migraines. Tension headaches are the most common type of headache and are often caused by stress or tension in the neck and shoulders. Cluster headaches are a less common type of headache that often occurs in cycles and can be very painful. Migraines are a severe type of headache that is often accompanied by other symptoms, such as sensitivity to light and sound, nausea, and vomiting.

How can acupressure help with headaches and migraines?

Acupressure is a natural therapy that involves applying pressure to specific points on the body to promote healing and well-being. Acupressure works by stimulating the body's natural healing mechanisms and promoting the flow of energy or Qi throughout the body. By applying pressure to specific points on the body, acupressure can help to relieve tension and pain, reduce inflammation, and promote relaxation. Here are some of the most commonly used acupressure points for headache and migraine relief:

1. LI4: Located in the fleshy webbing between the thumb and index finger, LI4 is commonly used to alleviate headaches and promote overall well-being. Applying pressure to LI4 can help to promote circulation and reduce stress, which can alleviate headaches.

2. GB20: Located at the base of the skull, in the hollows on either side of the neck, GB20 is commonly used to alleviate headaches and promote relaxation. Applying pressure to GB20 can help to promote circulation and reduce tension, which can alleviate headaches.

3. Yintang: Located between the eyebrows, Yintang is commonly used to alleviate headaches and promote relaxation. Applying pressure to Yintang can help to reduce stress and promote emotional balance, which can alleviate headaches.

4. GB21: Located on the top of the shoulders, GB21 is commonly used to alleviate headaches and promote relaxation. Applying pressure to GB21

can help to reduce tension in the neck and shoulders, which can alleviate headaches.

5. UB10: Located at the base of the skull, between the two vertical neck muscles, UB10 is commonly used to alleviate headaches and promote relaxation. Applying pressure to UB10 can help to reduce tension and promote circulation, which can alleviate headaches.

6. ST36: Located on the lower leg, about four finger widths below the kneecap, ST36 is commonly used to alleviate headaches and promote overall well-being. Applying pressure to ST36 can help to promote circulation and reduce tension, which can alleviate headaches.

How to apply acupressure for headaches and migraines?

To apply acupressure for headaches and migraines, it is best to sit or lie down in a comfortable position. Using your fingers or a small acupressure tool, apply firm pressure to the selected points for several minutes, breathing deeply and focusing on relaxation. You can repeat this process several times throughout the day or as needed to alleviate symptoms.

It is important to note that acupressure is not a substitute for medical treatment, and it is important to consult with a healthcare professional if you experience chronic or severe headaches or migraines.

Allergies and Sinus Issues

Allergies and sinus issues are common conditions that can cause discomfort and affect daily life. Traditional medicine treatments for allergies and sinus issues often include over-the-counter medications or prescription drugs. However, more and more people are turning to natural remedies like acupressure to alleviate their symptoms. In this article, we will explore how acupressure can be used to manage allergies and sinus issues.

What are allergies and sinus issues?

Allergies are a common condition that occurs when the immune system overreacts to a substance, such as pollen or pet dander. Allergies can cause symptoms such as sneezing, runny nose, itchy eyes, and skin rashes. Sinus issues are another common condition that occurs when the sinuses become inflamed or infected, causing symptoms such as nasal congestion, sinus pressure, and headache.

How can acupressure help with allergies and sinus issues?

Acupressure is a natural therapy that involves applying pressure to specific points on the body to promote healing and well-being. Acupressure works by stimulating the body's natural healing mechanisms and promoting the flow of energy or Qi throughout the body. By applying pressure to specific points on the body, acupressure can help to relieve congestion, reduce inflammation, and promote relaxation. Here are some of the most commonly used acupressure points for allergies and sinus issues:

1. LI20: Located on either side of the nose, at the base of the nostrils, LI20 is commonly used to alleviate sinus congestion and promote nasal drainage. Applying pressure to LI20 can help to stimulate the sinuses and promote drainage.

2. UB2: Located on the inside corner of the eyebrow, near the bridge of the nose, UB2 is commonly used to alleviate sinus congestion and promote relaxation. Applying pressure to UB2 can help to promote circulation and reduce tension in the sinuses.

3. LI4: Located in the fleshy webbing between the thumb and index finger, LI4 is commonly used to alleviate allergy symptoms and promote overall well-being. Applying pressure to LI4 can help to promote circulation and reduce inflammation, which can alleviate allergy symptoms.

4. GB20: Located at the base of the skull, in the hollows on either side of the neck, GB20 is commonly used to alleviate sinus congestion and promote relaxation. Applying pressure to GB20 can help to promote circulation and reduce tension in the neck and shoulders, which can alleviate sinus pressure.

5. Yintang: Located between the eyebrows, Yintang is commonly used to alleviate allergy symptoms and promote relaxation. Applying pressure to Yintang can help to reduce stress and promote emotional balance, which can alleviate allergy symptoms.

How to apply acupressure for allergies and sinus issues?

To apply acupressure for allergies and sinus issues, it is best to sit or lie down in a comfortable position. Using your fingers or a small acupressure tool, apply firm pressure to the selected points for several minutes, breathing deeply and focusing on relaxation. You can repeat this process several times throughout the day or as needed to alleviate symptoms.

It is important to note that acupressure is not a substitute for medical treatment, and it is important to consult with a healthcare professional if you experience chronic or severe allergies or sinus issues.

Joint and Muscle Pain

Joint and muscle pain can be caused by a variety of factors, including injury, overuse, arthritis, and inflammation. Traditional treatments for joint and muscle pain often involve pain medication and physical therapy, but more and more people are turning to natural remedies like acupressure to manage their symptoms. In this article, we will explore how acupressure can be used to alleviate joint and muscle pain.

What is acupressure?

Acupressure is a natural therapy that involves applying pressure to specific points on the body to promote healing and well-being. Acupressure works by stimulating the body's natural healing mechanisms and promoting the flow of energy or Qi throughout the body. By applying pressure to specific points on the body, acupressure can help to relieve pain, reduce inflammation, and promote relaxation.

How can acupressure help with joint and muscle pain?

Acupressure can be used to manage joint and muscle pain in a number of ways. First, acupressure can help to reduce inflammation, which is a common cause of joint pain. By applying pressure to specific points on the body, acupressure can help to promote the flow of blood and lymphatic fluid, which can reduce inflammation and promote healing.

Second, acupressure can help to relieve tension in the muscles, which can alleviate muscle pain. By applying pressure to specific points on the body, acupressure can help to promote relaxation and reduce tension in the muscles.

Third, acupressure can help to promote the flow of Qi, which is believed to be a vital energy that flows through the body. When the flow of Qi is blocked or disrupted, it can cause pain and discomfort. By applying pressure to specific points on the body, acupressure can help to promote the flow of Qi, which can alleviate pain and promote healing.

Here are some of the most commonly used acupressure points for joint and muscle pain:

1. GB34: Located on the outside of the lower leg, just below the knee, GB34 is commonly used to alleviate knee pain and promote overall well-being. Applying pressure to GB34 can help to promote circulation and reduce inflammation, which can alleviate knee pain.

2. LI4: Located in the fleshy webbing between the thumb and index finger, LI4 is commonly used to alleviate hand and wrist pain. Applying pressure to LI4 can help to promote circulation and reduce tension in the hand and wrist muscles.

3. GB20: Located at the base of the skull, in the hollows on either side of the neck, GB20 is commonly used to alleviate neck and shoulder pain. Applying pressure to GB20 can help to promote circulation and reduce tension in the neck and shoulder muscles.

4. BL60: Located on the outside of the ankle, behind the ankle bone, BL60 is commonly used to alleviate ankle and foot pain. Applying pressure to BL60 can help to promote circulation and reduce inflammation, which can alleviate ankle and foot pain.

5. CV6: Located two finger-widths below the belly button, CV6 is commonly used to alleviate abdominal pain and promote digestive health. Applying pressure to CV6 can help to promote the flow of Qi in the digestive system, which can alleviate abdominal pain.

How to apply acupressure for joint and muscle pain?

To apply acupressure for joint and muscle pain, it is best to sit or lie down in a comfortable position. Using your fingers or a small acupressure tool, apply firm pressure to the selected points for several minutes, breathing deeply and focusing on relaxation. You can repeat this process several times throughout the day or as needed to alleviate symptoms.

It is important to note that acupressure is not a substitute for medical treatment, and

Chapter Nine

Self-Acupressure Techniques

Acupressure is a natural therapy that involves applying pressure to specific points on the body to promote healing and well-being. Acupressure is often used to manage pain, reduce stress, and promote relaxation. While acupressure can be performed by a trained professional, it is also possible to perform self-acupressure techniques at home. In this article, we will explore some of the most effective self-acupressure techniques.

What is self-acupressure?

Self-acupressure is a natural therapy that involves applying pressure to specific points on the body to promote healing and well-being. Self-acupressure is a safe and effective way to manage pain, reduce stress, and promote relaxation. By applying pressure to specific points on the body, self-acupressure can help to promote the flow of energy or Qi throughout the body, which can alleviate pain and promote healing.

How to perform self-acupressure?

Performing self-acupressure is relatively easy and can be done at home. Here are some of the most effective self-acupressure techniques:

1. Hand technique: The hand technique involves applying pressure to specific points on the hands. To perform the hand technique, simply locate the point on the hand that corresponds to the area of the body where you

are experiencing pain or discomfort. Apply firm pressure to the point for several minutes, breathing deeply and focusing on relaxation.

2. Foot technique: The foot technique involves applying pressure to specific points on the feet. To perform the foot technique, simply locate the point on the foot that corresponds to the area of the body where you are experiencing pain or discomfort. Apply firm pressure to the point for several minutes, breathing deeply and focusing on relaxation.

3. Ear technique: The ear technique involves applying pressure to specific points on the ears. To perform the ear technique, simply locate the point on the ear that corresponds to the area of the body where you are experiencing pain or discomfort. Apply firm pressure to the point for several minutes, breathing deeply and focusing on relaxation.

4. Body technique: The body technique involves applying pressure to specific points on the body. To perform the body technique, simply locate the point on the body that corresponds to the area of the body where you are experiencing pain or discomfort. Apply firm pressure to the point for several minutes, breathing deeply and focusing on relaxation.

Here are some of the most effective self-acupressure points:

5. LI4: Located in the fleshy webbing between the thumb and index finger, LI4 is commonly used to alleviate hand and wrist pain. Applying pressure to LI4 can help to promote circulation and reduce tension in the hand and wrist muscles.

6. GB20: Located at the base of the skull, in the hollows on either side of the neck, GB20 is commonly used to alleviate neck and shoulder pain. Applying pressure to GB20 can help to promote circulation and reduce tension in the neck and shoulder muscles.

7. CV6: Located two finger-widths below the belly button, CV6 is commonly used to alleviate abdominal pain and promote digestive health. Applying pressure to CV6 can help to promote the flow of Qi in the digestive system, which can alleviate abdominal pain.

8. SP6: Located on the inside of the leg, just above the ankle, SP6 is commonly used to alleviate menstrual cramps and promote overall well-being. Applying pressure to SP6 can help to promote circulation and reduce tension in the leg muscles.

It is important to note that self-acupressure is not a substitute for medical treatment, and individuals should consult with a healthcare professional before using acupressure to manage any health condition. In addition, it is important to use proper techniques and to apply pressure with care, as applying too much pressure

Creating a Daily Routine

Acupressure is a natural therapy that can help to promote healing and well-being. While acupressure can be performed by a trained professional, it is also possible to perform self-acupressure techniques at home. To get the most out of acupressure, it is important to create a daily routine that incorporates these techniques into your daily life. In this article, we will explore some tips for creating a daily routine that incorporates acupressure.

Why create a daily routine?

Creating a daily routine that incorporates acupressure can be a powerful tool for promoting healing and well-being. By performing acupressure techniques on a daily basis, you can help to promote the flow of energy or Qi throughout your body, which can alleviate pain and promote healing.

In addition, creating a daily routine can help you to stay focused and on track with your health goals.

Tips for creating a daily routine:

1. Start small: When creating a daily routine, it is important to start small and build from there. Begin by incorporating one or two acupressure techniques into your routine, and gradually add more as you become more comfortable with the techniques.

2. Set aside time: To make acupressure a part of your daily routine, it is important to set aside time each day to perform these techniques. This can be as little as five or ten minutes a day, but it is important to be consistent.

3. Find a quiet space: When performing acupressure, it is important to find a quiet space where you can relax and focus on the technique. This can be a quiet room in your home, or even a peaceful spot outdoors.

4. Use visualization: Visualization can be a powerful tool for promoting healing and well-being. As you perform acupressure techniques, visualize the flow of energy or Qi throughout your body, and imagine the healing power of this energy.

5. Focus on relaxation: Acupressure techniques are most effective when performed in a state of relaxation. As you perform these techniques, focus on deep breathing and relaxing your body.

6. Make it a habit: Creating a daily routine takes time and effort, but it is important to make acupressure a habit. By incorporating these techniques into your daily routine, you can promote healing and well-being on a regular basis.

Here are some tips for incorporating acupressure into your daily routine:

7. Perform acupressure techniques in the morning: Performing acupressure techniques in the morning can help to promote energy and focus throughout the day.

8. Perform acupressure techniques before bed: Performing acupressure techniques before bed can help to promote relaxation and restful sleep.

9. Perform acupressure techniques during breaks: If you work at a desk or spend long periods of time sitting, taking breaks to perform acupressure techniques can help to promote circulation and alleviate tension in the muscles.

10. Use acupressure to manage stress: Acupressure techniques can be a powerful tool for managing stress. By incorporating acupressure into your daily routine, you can promote relaxation and reduce stress levels.

11. Use acupressure to manage pain: Acupressure techniques can be effective in managing pain. By incorporating these techniques into your daily routine, you can alleviate pain and promote healing.

Partner Acupressure

Acupressure is a natural therapy that involves applying pressure to specific points on the body to promote healing and well-being. While acupressure can be performed by a trained professional or through self-acupressure techniques, it is also possible to perform partner acupressure with a partner or loved one. In this article, we will explore what partner acupressure is, how it works, and some techniques for performing partner acupressure.

What is partner acupressure?

Partner acupressure is a form of acupressure that involves applying pressure to specific points on your partner's body to promote healing and relaxation. Unlike other forms of acupressure, partner acupressure involves working together with your partner to achieve relaxation and healing.

How does partner acupressure work?

Partner acupressure works by promoting the flow of energy or Qi throughout the body. When performed correctly, partner acupressure can help to alleviate tension, reduce stress levels, and promote relaxation. In addition, partner acupressure can be a powerful tool for improving communication and building trust in a relationship.

Techniques for performing partner acupressure:

1. Shoulder and neck acupressure: This technique involves applying pressure to the acupressure points located on the shoulders and neck. Begin by having your partner sit or lie down in a comfortable position. Use your fingertips to apply pressure to the acupressure points on the shoulders and neck, moving in a circular motion.

2. Foot acupressure: Foot acupressure is a powerful technique for promoting relaxation and reducing stress levels. Begin by having your partner sit or lie down in a comfortable position. Use your fingertips to apply pressure to the acupressure points on the feet, moving in a circular motion.

3. Hand acupressure: Hand acupressure can be a powerful tool for promoting relaxation and reducing stress levels. Begin by having your partner sit or lie down in a comfortable position. Use your fingertips to apply pressure to the acupressure points on the hands, moving in a circular motion.

4. Back acupressure: Back acupressure can be a powerful tool for reducing tension and promoting relaxation. Begin by having your partner lie face down on a comfortable surface. Use your fingertips to apply pressure to the acupressure points on the back, moving in a circular motion.

5. Head and face acupressure: Head and face acupressure can be a powerful tool for reducing stress levels and promoting relaxation. Begin by having your partner sit or lie down in a comfortable position. Use your fingertips to apply pressure to the acupressure points on the head and face, moving in a circular motion.

Acupressure Tools and Devices

Acupressure is an alternative therapy that involves applying pressure to specific points on the body to promote healing and relaxation. While acupressure can be performed by a trained professional or through self-acupressure techniques, there are also a variety of acupressure tools and devices available on the market. In this article, we will explore what acupressure tools and devices are, how they work, and some of the most popular types of acupressure tools and devices.

What are acupressure tools and devices?

Acupressure tools and devices are tools that can be used to perform acupressure on yourself or others. These tools are designed to help you apply pressure to specific points on the body more easily and effectively.

How do acupressure tools and devices work?

Acupressure tools and devices work by applying pressure to specific points on the body. When pressure is applied to these points, it can help to promote the flow of energy or Qi throughout the body, reduce tension, and promote relaxation. In addition, acupressure tools and devices can be a useful tool for individuals who have difficulty reaching certain areas of the body, such as the back or feet.

Types of acupressure tools and devices:

1. Acupressure mat: An acupressure mat is a mat that is covered in small plastic spikes or needles that are designed to stimulate acupressure points on the body. To use an acupressure mat, simply lie down on the mat and allow the spikes to apply pressure to your back, neck, and other areas of the body.

2. Acupressure ball: An acupressure ball is a small ball that is designed to be rolled over acupressure points on the body. To use an acupressure ball, simply apply pressure to the ball and roll it over the area where you want to stimulate acupressure points.

3. Acupressure ring: An acupressure ring is a small ring that is designed to apply pressure to specific acupressure points on the fingers. To use an acupressure ring, simply slide it onto your finger and move it up and down to stimulate acupressure points.

4. Acupressure pillow: An acupressure pillow is a pillow that is designed to stimulate acupressure points on the neck and shoulders. To use an acupressure pillow, simply lie down on the pillow and allow it to apply pressure to the acupressure points on your neck and shoulders.

5. Acupressure strap: An acupressure strap is a strap that is designed to apply pressure to acupressure points on the back. To use an acupressure strap, simply wrap it around your back and pull it tight to apply pressure to the acupressure points.

Chapter Ten

Integrating Acupressure into Your Life

Integrating Acupressure into Your Life

Acupressure is an ancient healing technique that has been used for thousands of years to promote relaxation, relieve pain, and improve overall health. It involves applying pressure to specific points on the body, known as acupoints, to stimulate the flow of energy or "chi" throughout the body. With the rise of interest in natural healing methods, more people are turning to acupressure as a way to complement conventional medicine or as an alternative therapy. Below we will explore how to integrate acupressure into your life for better physical, mental, and emotional health.

Learning the Basics

The first step in integrating acupressure into your life is to learn the basics. You can start by reading books, attending workshops or online classes, or consulting a licensed acupuncturist or acupressure therapist. Understanding the meridian system, acupoints, and techniques used in acupressure will help you to effectively apply it to your daily routine.

Set Realistic Goals

Acupressure is a safe and effective method of healing, but it is important to set realistic goals for yourself. It may take some time to see the results, especially if you are dealing with chronic or long-standing health issues.

Start with small, manageable goals, and gradually increase the amount of time you spend on acupressure each day.

Create a Daily Routine

Integrating acupressure into your daily routine is a great way to make it a regular part of your life. You can start by setting aside a few minutes each day to practice acupressure on yourself. Choose a time that works best for you, such as before bedtime, in the morning, or during your lunch break.

Practice Self-Acupressure

Self-acupressure is a convenient and easy way to integrate acupressure into your life. You can apply pressure to specific acupoints on your body using your fingers or a device. Self-acupressure can help to relieve stress, promote relaxation, and improve overall health. It is also a great way to treat minor ailments such as headaches, muscle pain, and digestive issues.

Use Acupressure in Combination with Other Therapies

Acupressure can be used in combination with other therapies such as massage, yoga, or meditation to enhance the healing process. These complementary therapies can help to promote relaxation, relieve stress, and improve overall health.

Seek Professional Help When Needed

While acupressure is generally safe, it is important to seek professional help when needed. If you have a serious medical condition or are taking medication, it is important to consult with your healthcare provider before using acupressure as a complementary therapy. Licensed acupuncturists and acupressure therapists can also provide guidance on how to effectively integrate acupressure into your life.

Experiment with Different Techniques and Tools

There are a variety of acupressure techniques and tools that you can use to enhance your practice. Experimenting with different techniques and tools can help you to find what works best for you. Some common tools include acupressure mats, rollers, and balls.

Stay Consistent

Consistency is key when it comes to integrating acupressure into your life. It may take some time to see the results, but staying consistent with your practice can help you to achieve better physical, mental, and emotional health.

Combining Acupressure with Other Therapies

Combining Acupressure with Other Therapies

Acupressure is a traditional healing practice that involves the use of finger pressure on specific points along the body's meridian lines to promote health and well-being. This technique has been used for centuries to treat a wide range of physical and emotional ailments. In recent years, acupressure has gained popularity in Western countries as an alternative and complementary therapy to conventional medical treatments. Many people are now exploring the benefits of combining acupressure with other therapies to enhance its effects and achieve better health outcomes. Below we will explore the ways in which acupressure can be combined with other therapies to promote health and well-being.

Acupressure can be combined with various other therapies, including massage, acupuncture, aromatherapy, and meditation. Massage and acupressure share some similarities in that both involve the use of touch to manipulate the body's soft tissues. Massage can help to loosen tight muscles, improve circulation, and release tension. When combined with acupressure, massage can enhance the effects of acupressure by promoting relaxation and improving the flow of qi, or energy, in the body. Massage can be particularly useful for treating conditions such as back pain, neck pain, and headaches, which often involve muscular tension.

Acupuncture and acupressure are two related therapies that share the same principles of Traditional Chinese Medicine. Acupuncture involves the insertion of thin needles into specific acupoints to stimulate the body's natural healing mechanisms. Acupressure, on the other hand, uses finger pressure to stimulate the same acupoints. When combined, these two therapies can be very effective in treating a wide range of conditions, from chronic pain to digestive disorders to emotional imbalances. Acupuncture and acupressure can be used in combination to achieve better pain relief and faster healing.

Aromatherapy involves the use of essential oils extracted from plants to promote physical and emotional well-being. Essential oils can be used in massage, added to bath water, or inhaled through a diffuser. When combined with acupressure, aromatherapy can enhance the relaxation and stress-reducing effects of acupressure. Essential oils such as lavender, chamomile, and peppermint are particularly useful for promoting relaxation and reducing stress.

Meditation is a practice that involves quieting the mind and focusing on the present moment. Meditation can be used to promote relaxation, reduce stress, and improve overall health and well-being. When combined with acupressure, meditation can enhance the effects of acupressure by promoting a deeper state of relaxation and increasing the flow of qi in the body. Meditation can also be useful for promoting mental clarity and emotional balance.

Other therapies that can be combined with acupressure include yoga, tai chi, and qigong. These practices all involve movements and postures that promote the flow of qi in the body. When combined with acupressure, these practices can enhance the effects of acupressure by promoting greater physical and emotional balance.

When combining acupressure with other therapies, it is important to seek guidance from a qualified practitioner who can provide personalized advice and support. A qualified acupressure practitioner can help to identify which therapies are most appropriate for your individual needs and can provide guidance on how to use these therapies safely and effectively.

Acupressure in the Workplace

Acupressure is a powerful tool that can be used to relieve stress and promote relaxation in many settings, including the workplace. The technique involves applying pressure to specific points on the body, which helps to release tension, reduce pain, and improve circulation. Acupressure can be performed by a trained practitioner, or it can be self-administered using various tools and techniques.

In the workplace, stress and tension can be a common problem for employees. Long hours, tight deadlines, and high-pressure situations can take a toll on both physical and mental health. Fortunately, acupressure can be a useful tool for managing stress and promoting well-being in the workplace.

One of the most common ways that acupressure is used in the workplace is through chair massage. This technique involves applying pressure to specific points on the back, neck, and shoulders while the individual is seated in a specially designed chair. Chair massage is a great way to relieve tension and promote relaxation in a short amount of time, making it a popular choice for busy workplaces.

Another way that acupressure can be used in the workplace is through the use of acupressure mats. These mats are covered in small plastic spikes that apply pressure to specific points on the body when laid on. Using an acupressure mat for just a few minutes a day can help to reduce tension and promote relaxation, making it a great tool for busy professionals who don't have a lot of time to devote to self-care.

In addition to chair massage and acupressure mats, there are many other ways that acupressure can be integrated into the workplace. Some companies offer regular yoga or meditation classes for employees, which can help to reduce stress and promote well-being. Others may provide access to trained acupressure practitioners who can offer individualized sessions to employees who need them.

There are also many simple acupressure techniques that individuals can use on their own in the workplace. For example, simply pressing the point between the thumb and index finger for a few minutes can help to relieve tension and reduce stress. Similarly, applying pressure to the point just below the base of the skull can help to relieve neck and shoulder tension.

It's important to note that while acupressure can be a useful tool for managing stress and promoting well-being in the workplace, it should not be used as a substitute for medical treatment. If an individual is experiencing chronic pain or other symptoms, they should seek medical attention from a qualified healthcare provider.

Acupressure for Athletes and Fitness Enthusiasts

Acupressure is a natural healing technique that can benefit athletes and fitness enthusiasts by promoting physical wellness, boosting energy, and reducing the risk of injuries. Acupressure, a form of Traditional Chinese Medicine, involves applying pressure to specific points on the body to stimulate the flow of Qi or energy. This therapy has been used for thousands of years to treat various conditions and promote overall health and wellness.

One of the most significant benefits of acupressure for athletes is its ability to improve circulation and reduce pain. By applying pressure to specific points on the body, acupressure can help to increase blood flow and reduce inflammation. This can be especially beneficial for athletes who are recovering from an injury or are experiencing muscle soreness after a workout.

Acupressure can also help to boost energy levels and promote mental clarity. By stimulating certain pressure points on the body, acupressure can help to improve focus and concentration, which can be especially useful for athletes who need to stay alert and attentive during a competition or training session.

Another benefit of acupressure is its ability to help reduce stress and anxiety. This therapy can help to calm the mind and reduce tension, which can be especially beneficial for athletes who are dealing with pre-competition nerves or who are experiencing stress related to training or competition.

In addition to its many physical and mental benefits, acupressure can also be used to promote better sleep. By stimulating specific pressure points on the body, acupressure can help to calm the mind and promote relaxation, which can lead to a more restful and rejuvenating night's sleep.

Athletes can use acupressure in several ways to promote physical and mental wellness. One way to incorporate acupressure into your routine is by visiting a licensed acupressure practitioner. During a session, the practitioner will apply pressure to specific points on your body, helping to promote physical and mental wellness.

Alternatively, athletes can also use self-acupressure techniques to promote wellness. There are many acupressure points on the body that can be stimulated through self-massage or with the use of acupressure tools such as balls or rollers. By incorporating self-acupressure into your routine, you can benefit from the many physical and mental benefits of this therapy on a regular basis.

Another way to incorporate acupressure into your life is by combining it with other therapies. Many athletes use acupressure in conjunction with other therapies such as massage, chiropractic care, or physical therapy to promote healing and overall wellness.

Finally, acupressure can also be used in the workplace to promote wellness and reduce stress. Many companies are now offering acupressure sessions to their employees as a way to promote physical and mental wellness and reduce stress levels in the workplace.

Chapter Eleven

Precautions and Contraindications

Acupressure is a traditional Chinese medicine technique that involves applying pressure to specific points on the body. While it can be a safe and effective form of therapy for many people, there are some precautions and contraindications to consider before trying acupressure.

One of the most important precautions to keep in mind is that acupressure should not be used as a substitute for medical care. If you have a serious or chronic health condition, it's important to speak with your healthcare provider before trying acupressure or any other form of complementary therapy.

Additionally, acupressure should not be used as a substitute for emergency medical care. If you experience a sudden or severe symptom, such as chest pain or difficulty breathing, seek immediate medical attention.

Certain conditions and situations may also make acupressure less safe or effective. For example, acupressure should not be used on open wounds or areas of the skin that are inflamed, infected, or otherwise irritated. If you have a skin condition such as eczema or psoriasis, it's important to avoid applying pressure to affected areas.

Pregnant women should also exercise caution when using acupressure, particularly on points that are known to stimulate the uterus. Some acupressure points are contraindicated during pregnancy, as they may cause contractions or other adverse effects. If you are pregnant, it's important to speak with your healthcare provider before trying acupressure or any other form of complementary therapy.

People with certain health conditions may also need to avoid or modify certain acupressure techniques. For example, if you have a bleeding disorder or are taking blood-thinning medications, applying pressure to certain points may increase the risk of bleeding. Similarly, if you have a heart condition or high blood pressure, some acupressure techniques may need to be modified or avoided.

It's also important to use caution when applying pressure to certain points on the body. For example, some points are located near major blood vessels or nerves, and applying too much pressure in these areas can be dangerous. Additionally, applying pressure to the wrong point can cause pain or other adverse effects.

If you are new to acupressure, it's a good idea to work with a trained practitioner who can help you identify safe and effective points to use. They can also help you learn proper techniques for applying pressure, and can monitor your progress to ensure that you are using acupressure safely and effectively.

When to Avoid Acupressure

Acupressure is a holistic therapy that has been used for centuries to promote healing, relaxation, and overall wellbeing. It involves applying pressure to specific points on the body to release tension and increase energy flow. While acupressure is generally considered safe and non-invasive, there are certain situations where it may not be appropriate or advisable. Below we will explore some of the instances where acupressure should be avoided.

Firstly, acupressure should be avoided in cases of acute injury or trauma, such as a broken bone, severe sprain or strain, or fresh wound. Applying pressure to these areas can exacerbate the injury and lead to further damage. Instead, it is important to seek immediate medical attention and follow the appropriate treatment plan recommended by a healthcare professional.

Secondly, acupressure should be avoided in certain medical conditions or situations. For example, if a person has a bleeding disorder or is taking blood-thinning medication, applying pressure to specific points can increase the risk of bleeding. Similarly, people with skin conditions such as eczema or psoriasis may experience irritation or further inflammation when pressure is applied to affected areas.

Pregnant women should also exercise caution when it comes to acupressure. While certain acupressure points may be helpful during pregnancy, others can stimulate the uterus and potentially induce labor or cause complications. It is important for pregnant women to consult with their healthcare provider before trying acupressure and to only receive treatment from a qualified practitioner.

People with certain medical devices, such as pacemakers or insulin pumps, should also avoid acupressure. Applying pressure to certain points can interfere with the function of these devices and potentially cause harm. It is important to consult with a healthcare provider before trying acupressure if you have a medical device.

Additionally, acupressure should be avoided in cases of fever, infectious disease, or acute illness. Stimulating specific points can increase circulation and energy flow, which can potentially exacerbate these conditions. It is important to rest and allow the body to heal during these times, and to seek appropriate medical treatment if necessary.

Finally, it is important to note that acupressure should not be used as a substitute for medical treatment. While it can be a helpful complementary therapy, it is not a replacement for medical care. If you have a medical condition or concern, it is important to seek guidance from a healthcare provider and to follow their recommended treatment plan.

Safety Tips and Guidelines

Acupressure is a non-invasive therapy that involves applying pressure to specific points on the body to stimulate healing and promote wellness. While it is generally considered safe, there are certain precautions and guidelines that should be followed to ensure safe and effective treatment.

One of the most important safety tips when performing acupressure is to ensure that you are using the correct pressure and technique for each point. Applying too much pressure or using incorrect technique can cause pain, bruising, or even injury. It is also important to use clean hands and tools when performing acupressure to prevent infection or the spread of illness.

Another important consideration when using acupressure is to avoid certain points during pregnancy. Some acupressure points are believed to stimulate contractions or induce labor, so it is important to consult with a healthcare provider before using acupressure during pregnancy.

In addition, acupressure should be avoided in certain medical conditions or situations. For example, if you have a broken bone or a serious injury, acupressure may exacerbate the condition or delay healing. Similarly, if you have a bleeding disorder or are taking blood-thinning medications, acupressure may increase the risk of bleeding or bruising.

It is also important to avoid using acupressure on areas of the body that are swollen, bruised, or injured. These areas may be more sensitive to pressure and may require more gentle techniques or a delay in treatment until the swelling or bruising has subsided.

When performing acupressure, it is important to pay attention to your body's response and to communicate any discomfort or pain to the therapist or healthcare provider. If you experience any unexpected or severe side effects, such as dizziness, nausea, or difficulty breathing, seek medical attention immediately.

In addition to following these safety tips, there are certain guidelines that can help to ensure safe and effective acupressure treatment. These include:

Always start with gentle pressure and gradually increase as needed.

Use a comfortable, stable position when performing acupressure to prevent strain or injury.

Focus on breathing deeply and slowly throughout the treatment to promote relaxation and reduce tension.

Take breaks as needed to prevent overstimulation or fatigue.

Use acupressure as part of a comprehensive treatment plan, including healthy lifestyle habits, exercise, and proper nutrition.

Seeking Professional Help

Acupressure is a form of alternative medicine that involves the application of pressure to specific points on the body to alleviate pain, promote relaxation, and improve overall well-being. While it is generally safe for most people to perform acupressure on themselves, seeking professional help is sometimes necessary to ensure the best results and to avoid potential risks.

When seeking professional help with acupressure, the first step is to find a qualified practitioner. This may involve researching acupressure clinics in your area or seeking recommendations from trusted friends or healthcare providers. It is important to choose a practitioner who is certified and experienced in acupressure techniques, and who has a good reputation for providing safe and effective treatment.

Once you have found a qualified practitioner, the next step is to schedule a consultation. During this consultation, the practitioner will ask about your medical history, any current health conditions, and any medications or supplements you are taking. They will also ask about your symptoms and any pain or discomfort you are experiencing.

Based on this information, the practitioner will then develop a treatment plan tailored to your individual needs. This may involve a combination of acupressure techniques, as well as other complementary therapies such as acupuncture, herbal medicine, or dietary and lifestyle recommendations.

During the treatment session, the practitioner will apply pressure to specific acupressure points on your body using their hands, fingers, or other specialized tools. The pressure applied may vary depending on your individual needs and the specific points being targeted.

It is important to communicate openly with the practitioner throughout the treatment session. If you experience any discomfort or pain, or if you have any concerns about the treatment, it is important to speak up and let the practitioner know. They can adjust the pressure or technique as needed to ensure your comfort and safety.

Following the treatment session, the practitioner may provide additional recommendations for self-care and follow-up appointments. They may also provide guidance on how to incorporate acupressure into your daily routine for optimal results.

While seeking professional help for acupressure can be beneficial, it is important to keep in mind that this form of therapy is not a substitute for medical care. If you are experiencing serious or chronic health conditions, or if you have concerns about your overall health and well-being, it is important to seek guidance from a qualified healthcare provider.

Additionally, while acupressure is generally safe for most people, there are certain situations where it may be contraindicated. For example, acupressure should not be performed on areas of the body that are bruised, swollen, or inflamed, or on areas of the body where there is an infection or open wound. It should also be avoided during pregnancy, and should be used with caution in people with certain health conditions such as diabetes or high blood pressure.

Chapter Twelve

Becoming an Acupressure Practitioner

Acupressure is a traditional Chinese medicine practice that involves applying pressure to specific points on the body to stimulate the flow of energy or "chi" and promote healing. While acupressure is often used as a self-care technique, some people may choose to become acupressure practitioners to help others improve their health and wellbeing.

To become an acupressure practitioner, one must first understand the principles and techniques of acupressure. This involves learning about the meridian system, pressure points, and the proper application of pressure. In addition, a deep understanding of anatomy, physiology, and pathology is necessary to effectively diagnose and treat imbalances in the body.

There are many ways to become an acupressure practitioner, including formal education and training programs, apprenticeships, and self-study. Formal education programs can range from short-term workshops to multi-year degree programs. These programs typically cover the theory and practice of acupressure, as well as related topics such as nutrition, herbal medicine, and bodywork.

Apprenticeships provide a more hands-on approach to learning acupressure. These programs involve working closely with a seasoned acupressure practitioner to gain practical experience and knowledge. While apprenticeships may be less formal than traditional education programs, they offer a more personalized learning experience and the opportunity to build relationships within the acupressure community.

Self-study is also a viable option for those interested in becoming acupressure practitioners. There are many books, online courses, and instructional videos available that can provide a solid foundation in acupressure theory and practice. However, self-study may not provide the same level of hands-on experience and feedback as formal education or apprenticeships.

In addition to learning the principles and techniques of acupressure, becoming a practitioner also requires developing strong interpersonal and communication skills. Practitioners must be able to listen to and understand their clients' needs and concerns, and communicate clearly and effectively about treatment options and progress.

Becoming an acupressure practitioner also involves developing a strong ethical foundation. Practitioners must adhere to professional standards of conduct and ensure that they are providing safe and effective care to their clients. This includes obtaining appropriate licensure and certifications, maintaining client confidentiality, and practicing within the scope of their training and expertise.

Training and Certification

Acupressure is a therapeutic technique that involves applying pressure on specific points on the body to stimulate the body's natural healing abilities. This technique has been used for thousands of years in traditional Chinese medicine and is gaining popularity in the Western world due to its effectiveness in treating a wide range of health conditions. Acupressure practitioners are highly skilled professionals who use this technique to improve the health and well-being of their clients.

To become an acupressure practitioner, it is essential to undergo comprehensive training and obtain certification from a reputable institution. The training and certification process ensures that practitioners have the necessary knowledge and skills to provide safe and effective treatment to their clients.

The first step in becoming an acupressure practitioner is to research and choose a reputable training program. It is important to select a program that is accredited by a recognized organization such as the National Certification Commission for Acupuncture and Oriental Medicine (NCCAOM). The training program should cover the theory and practical aspects of acupressure and provide hands-on experience in working with clients.

During the training, students will learn about the principles of acupressure, the meridian system, and the various pressure points on the body. They will also learn about the different techniques used in acupressure, including finger pressure, palm pressure, and elbow pressure. Additionally, students will learn about the proper application of pressure and the precautions and contraindications associated with acupressure.

In addition to the theoretical and practical training, students may also be required to complete a certain number of clinical hours under the supervision of a licensed acupressure practitioner. This will give them the opportunity to work with clients and gain hands-on experience in diagnosing and treating various health conditions.

Once the training is complete, the next step is to obtain certification. The certification process typically involves passing an exam that covers the theoretical and practical aspects of acupressure. The exam may be administered by a professional organization such as the NCCAOM or a state licensing board.

After obtaining certification, acupressure practitioners can start practicing independently or work under the supervision of a licensed acupuncturist or other healthcare provider. They may also choose to specialize in a particular area such as sports medicine, pain management, or women's health.

In addition to the initial training and certification, acupressure practitioners are also required to maintain their skills and knowledge through continuing education courses. These courses ensure that practitioners are up-to-date with the latest techniques and developments in acupressure and can provide the best possible care to their clients.

Building a Successful Practice

Acupressure is an ancient healing technique that has been used for thousands of years to relieve pain and promote healing. Today, it is still a popular and effective treatment for a wide range of conditions. Acupressure practitioners have the opportunity to build successful practices and help many people improve their health and well-being. Below we will explore some tips for building a successful acupressure practice.

The first step in building a successful acupressure practice is to gain a thorough understanding of the principles and techniques of acupressure. This includes knowledge of the meridian system, pressure points, and the proper application of pressure. In addition, practitioners should have an understanding of how acupressure can be used to treat specific conditions and promote overall wellness.

To gain this knowledge, practitioners may need to complete a comprehensive training program. There are many programs available, ranging from short courses to more extensive programs that can take several years to complete. Choosing the right program is an important step in building a successful practice.

Once a practitioner has gained a solid understanding of acupressure, they can begin to build their practice. One of the most important steps in building a successful practice is to establish a strong client base. This can be achieved through networking, marketing, and providing high-quality services.

Networking is an essential aspect of building a successful acupressure practice. Practitioners can network with other healthcare professionals, such as doctors and chiropractors, to build referral networks. They can also attend industry events and conferences to meet other practitioners and potential clients.

Marketing is another key component of building a successful practice. Practitioners can market their services through various channels, including social media, email marketing, and advertising. It is important to focus on the benefits of acupressure, such as pain relief, improved sleep, and reduced stress, when creating marketing materials.

Providing high-quality services is essential to building a successful acupressure practice. This means providing personalized care to each client, taking the time to understand their individual needs and concerns. It also means staying up to date with the latest techniques and research in the field of acupressure.

In addition to providing high-quality services, practitioners should also focus on building strong relationships with their clients. This means providing a comfortable and welcoming environment, being responsive to client needs and concerns, and following up with clients after their treatments.

Another important aspect of building a successful acupressure practice is maintaining a strong online presence. This includes having a website that is easy to navigate and provides information about the practitioner's services and expertise. It also means engaging with clients and potential clients through social media, email newsletters, and other online channels.

Finally, building a successful acupressure practice requires ongoing education and professional development. Practitioners should attend workshops, seminars, and other training opportunities to stay up to date with the latest techniques and research in the field. They should also seek out mentors and other experienced practitioners to learn from their expertise.

Ethical Considerations

Acupressure is an ancient healing technique that has been used for centuries to alleviate various ailments, promote wellness, and improve overall health. As acupressure becomes more popular in mainstream healthcare, it is essential to consider ethical considerations that practitioners and clients should be aware of.

Firstly, one of the essential ethical considerations in acupressure is informed consent. It is essential for acupressure practitioners to provide their clients with accurate information about the treatment, including the potential risks and benefits. Clients should be able to make informed decisions about their health, and practitioners should respect their choices. Additionally, practitioners should obtain written consent from clients before providing acupressure treatments.

Another important ethical consideration in acupressure is confidentiality. Clients trust practitioners with their personal health information, and practitioners should not disclose any information without their clients' consent. Practitioners should also maintain accurate and secure records and dispose of them appropriately once the treatment is complete.

Practitioners should also be aware of their professional boundaries and avoid engaging in any inappropriate behavior or relationships with their clients. Clients should be able to trust their practitioners, and practitioners should respect their clients' boundaries.

Furthermore, acupressure practitioners should respect cultural and individual differences among their clients. Clients come from diverse backgrounds and may have different beliefs and preferences. Practitioners should be aware of cultural differences and be respectful of clients' beliefs and values. They should also tailor their treatments to meet individual needs, preferences, and health conditions.

Another ethical consideration in acupressure is maintaining professional competence. Practitioners should pursue ongoing education and training to maintain their skills and knowledge. They should also be aware of their limitations and refer clients to other healthcare providers when necessary.

Lastly, acupressure practitioners should charge fair and reasonable fees for their services. They should be transparent about their fees and avoid charging excessively or taking advantage of their clients.

Chapter Thirteen

The Future of Acupressure

Acupressure is an ancient healing technique that has been used for thousands of years to treat various physical and mental ailments. It involves applying pressure to specific points on the body, known as acupoints, to stimulate the body's natural healing process. In recent years, acupressure has gained increasing popularity as a natural, non-invasive alternative to traditional medical treatments.

As we look to the future of acupressure, there are several exciting developments and trends to watch out for. One such trend is the integration of technology into acupressure practice. With the rise of wearable technology and the Internet of Things (IoT), it's now possible to track and monitor various health metrics, such as heart rate, sleep patterns, and stress levels. This information can be used to personalize acupressure treatments and improve their effectiveness.

Another trend in the future of acupressure is the growing interest in evidence-based research. While acupressure has been used for centuries to treat a variety of conditions, there is still a need for more scientific research to fully understand its mechanisms and effectiveness. As more research is conducted, we can expect to see more standardized acupressure protocols and a better understanding of how acupressure works on a physiological level.

One area where acupressure has shown promise is in the treatment of chronic pain. According to the National Institutes of Health (NIH), chronic pain affects an estimated 25 million adults in the United States alone. Acupressure has been shown to be an effective treatment for various types of chronic pain, including low back pain, neck pain, and arthritis. As the opioid epidemic continues to worsen, acupressure may become a more widely recognized alternative for pain management.

As the world becomes more aware of the importance of mental health, we can also expect to see a greater emphasis on the use of acupressure for mental health conditions. Acupressure has been shown to be effective in reducing symptoms of anxiety, depression, and stress, as well as improving overall mental well-being. With mental health becoming a more prominent issue in society, acupressure may become an increasingly popular complementary therapy for those seeking relief from mental health conditions.

Lastly, we can expect to see more integration of acupressure into mainstream healthcare. While acupressure has traditionally been seen as an alternative or complementary therapy, there is a growing recognition of its effectiveness and safety. As a result, we may see more acupressure clinics and practitioners working alongside traditional medical professionals to provide patients with a holistic approach to healthcare.

Emerging Research and Techniques

Acupressure is an ancient healing technique that has been used for thousands of years to promote health and wellbeing. It involves applying pressure to specific points on the body, known as acupoints, to stimulate the body's natural healing abilities. Acupressure has been used to treat a wide range of conditions, including pain, stress, anxiety, and digestive disorders.

Over the years, acupressure has gained popularity as an alternative therapy, and its effectiveness has been supported by emerging research. Below we will explore some of the latest research and techniques in acupressure.

One area of emerging research in acupressure is its effectiveness in treating chronic pain. Chronic pain is a widespread health problem that affects millions of people worldwide. It can be caused by various conditions, such as arthritis, fibromyalgia, and back pain. Acupressure has been shown to be effective in reducing pain and improving quality of life in people with chronic pain. One study found that acupressure was more effective than usual care in reducing pain intensity and disability in people with chronic low back pain. Another study showed that acupressure was effective in reducing pain and improving function in people with knee osteoarthritis.

Another area of research in acupressure is its potential role in treating anxiety and depression. Anxiety and depression are among the most common mental health disorders, affecting millions of people worldwide. Acupressure has been shown to be effective in reducing anxiety and depression symptoms in several studies. One study found that acupressure was effective in reducing anxiety symptoms in patients with coronary artery disease. Another study showed that acupressure was effective in reducing depression symptoms in people with depression.

In recent years, new techniques in acupressure have been developed to enhance its effectiveness. One such technique is called ear acupressure or auricular acupressure. This technique involves applying pressure to specific points on the ear to treat various conditions. Auricular acupressure has been shown to be effective in treating anxiety, pain, and addiction. Another technique is called laser acupressure, which involves using low-level laser therapy to stimulate acupoints. This technique has been shown to be effective in treating pain, inflammation, and wound healing.

In addition to new techniques, new technologies have also been developed to enhance the effectiveness of acupressure. One such technology is called the acupressure mat, which is a mat covered with thousands of small spikes that stimulate acupoints on the back. The acupressure mat has been shown to be effective in reducing pain, stress, and anxiety.

While acupressure is generally safe, there are some precautions and contraindications that should be considered. For example, acupressure should be avoided during pregnancy, in people with certain medical conditions, and in areas with broken skin or wounds. It is important to seek advice from a qualified acupressure practitioner before undergoing any treatment.

Acupressure in Modern Medicine

Acupressure is an ancient healing technique that has been practiced for thousands of years in China and other parts of Asia. It involves the application of pressure to specific points on the body, known as acupoints, to stimulate the body's natural healing processes and restore balance to the flow of energy, or chi. While traditionally used as a complementary or alternative therapy, acupressure is now gaining recognition in modern medicine for its potential benefits in pain management, stress reduction, and other areas of health and wellness.

One area where acupressure is gaining particular attention is in pain management. According to the National Institutes of Health (NIH), acupuncture and acupressure are effective for treating a variety of chronic pain conditions, including back pain, neck pain, osteoarthritis, and headaches. Acupressure has been shown to stimulate the release of endorphins, the body's natural pain relievers, and to block the transmission of pain signals to the brain. This makes it an attractive option for people who are looking for non-pharmacological approaches to pain management.

Acupressure is also gaining recognition for its potential benefits in stress reduction. In today's fast-paced world, stress is a major contributor to a wide range of health problems, including cardiovascular disease, depression, and anxiety. Acupressure has been shown to stimulate the release of oxytocin, a hormone that promotes relaxation and reduces stress, and to reduce levels of cortisol, a stress hormone that can contribute to a range of health problems. Studies have also shown that acupressure can help improve sleep quality and reduce symptoms of anxiety and depression.

Another area where acupressure is showing promise is in the treatment of digestive disorders. Acupressure has been used for centuries in Traditional Chinese Medicine to treat a variety of digestive issues, including constipation, diarrhea, and indigestion. It works by stimulating the body's natural digestive processes and promoting the flow of energy to the digestive organs. Studies have shown that acupressure can be effective in reducing symptoms of irritable bowel syndrome (IBS) and other digestive disorders.

Acupressure is also gaining recognition as a complementary therapy for cancer patients. It has been shown to reduce symptoms such as nausea, vomiting, and fatigue, which are common side effects of cancer treatment. Acupressure is thought to work by stimulating the release of endorphins and other natural pain relievers, as well as by promoting relaxation and reducing stress.

As acupressure gains recognition in modern medicine, new techniques and technologies are emerging that are making it easier for healthcare professionals to incorporate acupressure into their practices. One example is the use of acupressure mats, which are designed to stimulate acupoints on the back and neck to relieve pain and tension. Another example is the use of electroacupuncture, which involves the use of a small electric current to stimulate acupoints.

Despite its growing popularity in modern medicine, acupressure is not without its critics. Some healthcare professionals remain skeptical of its effectiveness, and there is a need for further research to fully understand its mechanisms of action and potential benefits. Additionally, as with any therapy, it is important to use acupressure safely and under the guidance of a trained professional.

Innovations in Acupressure Therapy

Acupressure, a form of alternative medicine, has been used for thousands of years to promote healing and well-being. This therapy involves applying pressure to specific points on the body, known as acupoints, to stimulate the body's natural healing mechanisms. While the basic principles of acupressure remain the same, there have been many innovations in recent years that have expanded the scope and effectiveness of this therapy. Below we will explore some of the latest innovations in acupressure therapy and their potential benefits.

One of the most exciting developments in acupressure therapy is the use of technology to enhance its effectiveness. For example, acupressure mats, also known as spike mats or nail mats, have become increasingly popular in recent years. These mats are covered in hundreds of small plastic spikes that are designed to apply pressure to acupoints in the back and neck. Users lie on the mat for 20-30 minutes each day to stimulate blood flow, reduce pain and stress, and promote relaxation. While there is limited scientific research on the effectiveness of acupressure mats, many users report significant improvements in their symptoms and well-being.

Another innovation in acupressure therapy is the use of electrical stimulation to enhance the effects of acupressure. Electrical stimulation involves the use of a small device that delivers low-frequency electrical impulses to the acupoints. This therapy is believed to stimulate the release of endorphins and other natural pain-relieving chemicals in the body. It is commonly used to treat chronic pain conditions such as fibromyalgia and back pain, as well as to promote relaxation and reduce stress.

In recent years, there has also been growing interest in the use of acupressure for cosmetic purposes. Facial acupressure, also known as acupressure facelift, involves applying pressure to specific points on the face to stimulate blood flow, reduce wrinkles and fine lines, and promote a more youthful appearance. This therapy is often used as a natural alternative to Botox and other cosmetic treatments that can be expensive and have potential side effects. While there is limited scientific evidence to support the effectiveness of facial acupressure, many people report noticeable improvements in their skin's appearance and texture after regular treatment.

Acupressure has also been used to support mental health and well-being, with recent innovations in this area focused on using acupressure to address specific mental health conditions. For example, Emotional Freedom Technique (EFT) is a form of acupressure therapy that is often used to treat anxiety, depression, and other mental health conditions. This therapy involves tapping on specific acupoints while focusing on specific thoughts or emotions. It is believed to release blockages in the body's energy system and promote emotional healing.

Another innovation in acupressure therapy is the use of auricular acupressure, also known as ear acupressure, to treat addiction and cravings. This therapy involves applying pressure to specific points on the ear that correspond to different organs and body systems. It is commonly used to support recovery from addiction to drugs, alcohol, and nicotine, as well as to reduce cravings and withdrawal symptoms.

Chapter Fourteen

Acupressure for Children and Teens

Acupressure, a traditional Chinese healing technique, has been used for centuries to promote health and wellness. It involves applying pressure to specific points on the body to stimulate the body's natural healing processes. While it's commonly used by adults, acupressure can also be a safe and effective treatment for children and teens. Below we will we'll explore the benefits of acupressure for children and teens and how it can be safely and effectively integrated into their healthcare.

Acupressure is a holistic approach to healing that is based on the belief that the body has an energy system made up of meridians, or channels, that flow through the body. These meridians correspond to different organs and systems in the body, and when they become blocked or imbalanced, it can lead to illness or disease. By applying pressure to specific points on the body, acupressure can help to stimulate the flow of energy and restore balance to the body.

One of the benefits of acupressure for children and teens is that it can help to relieve stress and anxiety. Children and teens today are often under a lot of pressure from school, extracurricular activities, and social media. This can lead to high levels of stress and anxiety, which can have a negative impact on their physical and emotional health. Acupressure can help to release tension and promote relaxation, which can reduce stress and anxiety levels.

Another benefit of acupressure for children and teens is that it can help to improve sleep quality. Sleep is essential for growth and development, but many children and teens struggle with sleep issues such as insomnia or sleep apnea. Acupressure can help to promote relaxation and reduce tension, which can lead to better sleep quality.

Acupressure can also be used to address specific health issues in children and teens. For example, it can be used to relieve symptoms of allergies, asthma, and digestive issues. It can also be used to reduce pain and inflammation associated with conditions such as arthritis and sports injuries.

It's important to note that while acupressure can be a safe and effective treatment for children and teens, it should always be performed by a trained and experienced practitioner. Children and teens have smaller and more delicate bodies than adults, so the pressure and duration of acupressure should be adjusted accordingly.

Parents should also be aware of any contraindications or precautions associated with acupressure. For example, certain points should be avoided during pregnancy or if the child has a bleeding disorder. A qualified acupressure practitioner will be able to assess the child's individual needs and ensure that the treatment is safe and appropriate.

In addition to professional acupressure treatment, there are also self-care techniques that children and teens can use at home to promote health and wellness. These can include simple techniques such as gentle massage or applying pressure to specific points on the body. It's important to teach children and teens how to perform these techniques safely and effectively.

Gentle Techniques for Kids

Acupressure is an ancient healing technique that has been used for centuries to treat various health issues. This practice involves applying pressure to specific points on the body, which are believed to correspond to different organs and systems in the body. While acupressure is often associated with adults, it can also be used to treat children and teenagers. Below we will explore gentle techniques for kids that can help them experience the benefits of acupressure.

Acupressure for children and teenagers is a safe and effective way to promote health and wellness. One of the main benefits of acupressure is that it can help to relieve stress and anxiety, which are common issues that children and teenagers may face. By applying pressure to specific points on the body, acupressure can help to calm the mind and relax the body, which can reduce feelings of stress and anxiety.

One of the most common acupressure techniques for children is called the "Belly Button Massage." This technique involves gently massaging the area around the belly button in a clockwise motion. This technique is believed to help with digestion, relieve constipation, and promote relaxation. To perform this technique, have your child lie down on their back and place your hand on their belly button. Gently massage the area in a clockwise motion for a few minutes.

Another gentle acupressure technique that can be used for children is called the "Ear Massage." This technique involves gently massaging the earlobe and the area behind the ear. This technique is believed to help with headaches, earaches, and other issues related to the head and neck. To perform this technique, have your child sit or lie down and gently massage their earlobe and the area behind the ear for a few minutes.

The "Heart Hug" technique is another gentle acupressure technique that can be used for children. This technique involves giving your child a gentle hug while placing your hand over their heart. This technique is believed to help with emotional issues, such as anxiety, depression, and grief. To perform this technique, simply give your child a gentle hug while placing your hand over their heart.

The "Rubbing the Soles of the Feet" technique is another gentle acupressure technique that can be used for children. This technique involves gently rubbing the soles of the feet, which is believed to help with sleep issues, anxiety, and digestive issues. To perform this technique, have your child sit down and gently rub the soles of their feet for a few minutes.

It's important to note that while acupressure is generally safe for children and teenagers, there are some precautions that should be taken. For example, certain acupressure points should be avoided during pregnancy or if your child has a specific medical condition. It's also important to be gentle when performing acupressure on children, as their bodies are more delicate than adults.

In addition to using acupressure techniques on their own, children can also benefit from receiving acupressure treatments from a trained practitioner. An acupressure practitioner can work with your child to develop a treatment plan that addresses their specific needs and concerns. They can also teach you and your child techniques that can be used at home to promote health and wellness.

Acupressure for Common Childhood Ailments

Acupressure is an alternative therapy that has been used for centuries to alleviate various health issues, including common childhood ailments. It involves applying pressure to specific points on the body to stimulate the body's natural healing abilities. Acupressure can be a safe and effective way to treat many conditions in children, as long as it is performed correctly and by a trained practitioner or under the guidance of a healthcare professional. Below we will discuss some of the common childhood ailments that can be treated with acupressure.

One of the most common childhood ailments is earaches. Earaches can be caused by many factors, including infections, allergies, or changes in air pressure. Acupressure can be used to relieve the pain associated with earaches. The pressure points for earaches are located on the hands and feet. To stimulate these points, gentle pressure is applied to the webbing between the thumb and index finger or the base of the pinky finger. Alternatively, pressure can be applied to the center of the foot, just below the second and third toes.

Another common childhood ailment is asthma. Asthma is a chronic respiratory condition that can cause wheezing, coughing, and difficulty breathing. Acupressure can be used to manage asthma symptoms and improve lung function. The pressure points for asthma are located on the upper back and chest. To stimulate these points, gentle pressure is applied to the space between the shoulder blades or just below the collarbone.

Acupressure can also be used to treat digestive problems in children. Common digestive problems in children include constipation, diarrhea, and stomachaches. The pressure points for digestive problems are located on the abdomen. To stimulate these points, gentle pressure is applied to the area just below the belly button or on the sides of the abdomen.

Another common childhood ailment is headaches. Headaches can be caused by a variety of factors, including stress, dehydration, and tension. Acupressure can be used to relieve headaches and promote relaxation. The pressure points for headaches are located on the head and neck. To stimulate these points, gentle pressure is applied to the temples or the base of the skull.

Bedwetting is another common childhood ailment that can be treated with acupressure. Bedwetting is the involuntary release of urine during sleep. The pressure points for bedwetting are located on the lower back and abdomen. To stimulate these points, gentle pressure is applied to the lower back or on the sides of the abdomen, just above the hip bone.

Acupressure can also be used to manage anxiety and promote relaxation in children. Anxiety is a common problem in children and can be caused by a variety of factors, including stress, trauma, and changes in routine. The pressure points for anxiety are located on the wrists and chest. To stimulate these points, gentle pressure is applied to the inside of the wrist or the center of the chest.

It is important to note that acupressure should not be used as a substitute for medical care. Parents should consult with a healthcare professional before using acupressure to treat their child's health problems. Acupressure can be used in conjunction with conventional medical treatments to provide additional relief and promote healing.

Promoting Healthy Development

Acupressure, an alternative therapy based on Traditional Chinese Medicine, has been increasingly used for promoting healthy development in children. Acupressure involves applying pressure to specific points on the body, known as acupoints, to stimulate the flow of Qi, the body's vital energy. This can help to balance the body's functions, alleviate symptoms, and promote overall health and well-being. Below we will explore how acupressure can be used to promote healthy development in children.

The use of acupressure for promoting healthy development in children is based on the idea that children's bodies are more sensitive and receptive to touch and that acupressure can help to enhance their physical, emotional, and cognitive development. Acupressure can be used for a wide range of childhood conditions, such as colic, teething, bedwetting, asthma, allergies, ADHD, and anxiety.

One of the main benefits of acupressure for children is its non-invasive nature. Acupressure can be used as a safe and gentle therapy for children of all ages, including infants and toddlers. It does not involve the use of drugs, needles, or invasive procedures, which can be stressful and traumatic for young children. Acupressure can also be easily incorporated into a child's daily routine and can be done at home, by parents or caregivers.

Acupressure can be used to promote healthy physical development in children by improving digestion, boosting immunity, and reducing pain and inflammation. Acupressure can help to stimulate the digestive system, which can be especially beneficial for children with digestive issues, such as colic and constipation. Acupressure can also help to boost the immune system, which can help to prevent and reduce the severity of illnesses, such as colds and flu. Acupressure can also help to reduce pain and inflammation, which can be beneficial for children with conditions such as arthritis, asthma, and allergies.

Acupressure can also be used to promote healthy emotional development in children. Acupressure can help to reduce anxiety and stress, which can be beneficial for children who are experiencing anxiety due to school, family issues, or other sources. Acupressure can also help to improve mood and increase feelings of well-being, which can be beneficial for children who are experiencing depression or other emotional issues.

Acupressure can also be used to promote healthy cognitive development in children. Acupressure can help to improve concentration, focus, and memory, which can be beneficial for children who are struggling with ADHD or other learning disabilities. Acupressure can also help to promote mental clarity and alertness, which can be beneficial for children who are experiencing brain fog or other cognitive issues.

When using acupressure for children, it is important to use gentle techniques that are appropriate for their age and developmental stage. Parents and caregivers should also be familiar with the acupoints that are safe and appropriate for children. Some acupoints, such as those on the face or neck, should be avoided in young children to prevent injury. It is also important to use acupressure in conjunction with other therapies, such as diet and lifestyle changes, to promote overall health and well-being.

Chapter Fifteen

Acupressure for Seniors

Acupressure is a traditional Chinese healing technique that has been used for thousands of years to promote health and well-being. It involves applying pressure to specific points on the body to stimulate the body's natural healing abilities. Acupressure is a safe and effective therapy that can be used by people of all ages, including seniors.

As we age, our bodies undergo various changes that can lead to a decline in health and well-being. Acupressure can help seniors to maintain their health and improve their quality of life by promoting better circulation, reducing pain and inflammation, boosting the immune system, and reducing stress and anxiety.

One of the most common health issues that seniors face is chronic pain, particularly in the joints and muscles. Acupressure can be an effective way to alleviate this pain by stimulating the body's natural pain-relieving mechanisms. By applying pressure to specific points on the body, acupressure can help to increase blood flow and reduce inflammation in the affected areas.

Another common issue that seniors face is poor circulation, which can lead to a range of health problems, including heart disease, stroke, and cognitive decline. Acupressure can help to improve circulation by stimulating the body's natural energy flow. By applying pressure to specific points on the body, acupressure can help to increase blood flow to the brain and other vital organs, improving their function and reducing the risk of age-related decline.

Stress and anxiety are also common issues that seniors face, particularly as they deal with the challenges of aging and changes in their social and family relationships. Acupressure can be an effective way to reduce stress and promote relaxation by stimulating the body's natural relaxation response. By applying pressure to specific points on the body, acupressure can help to activate the parasympathetic nervous system, which is responsible for promoting relaxation and reducing stress.

In addition to these general benefits, there are also specific acupressure points that can be particularly beneficial for seniors. For example, the point known as "Gallbladder 20" is located at the base of the skull and is believed to improve memory and cognitive function. The point known as "Kidney 1" is located on the sole of the foot and is believed to promote longevity and vitality.

There are also some special considerations that need to be taken into account when using acupressure with seniors. For example, the pressure applied during acupressure should be gentle and not too intense, as seniors' skin can be more delicate and sensitive than that of younger people. Seniors should also be monitored carefully for any adverse effects or reactions, and acupressure should be discontinued if any negative symptoms occur.

Adapting Techniques for Older Adults

Acupressure is a technique that has been used for centuries to treat a variety of ailments, including pain, stress, and insomnia. It is a non-invasive, safe, and effective way to promote healing and relaxation. Acupressure is particularly useful for seniors who may be more vulnerable to the side effects of medication and other invasive treatments. However, the technique may need to be adapted to suit the needs and abilities of older adults.

One of the main concerns when using acupressure with seniors is the risk of injury. Older adults may have fragile bones and delicate skin, which can be easily bruised or damaged. Therefore, it is important to use a gentle touch and apply pressure slowly and gradually. It is also essential to avoid applying pressure to areas that are painful or tender, as this can cause discomfort or exacerbate existing conditions.

Another important consideration when using acupressure with seniors is the positioning of the body. Older adults may have limited mobility and flexibility, which can make it difficult to access certain acupressure points. Therefore, it may be necessary to modify the position of the body or use pillows and cushions to provide support and comfort.

One way to adapt acupressure techniques for seniors is to focus on the hands and feet. These areas are often more accessible and less sensitive than other parts of the body. By applying pressure to specific points on the hands and feet, acupressure can help to relieve pain, reduce stress, and promote relaxation.

For example, applying pressure to the "hoku" point, located on the webbing between the thumb and index finger, can help to relieve headaches and neck pain. Similarly, pressing on the "yongquan" point, located on the sole of the foot, can help to reduce anxiety and promote better sleep.

Another way to adapt acupressure for seniors is to use a light touch. Gentle massage or tapping can be just as effective as deep pressure in promoting relaxation and easing pain. This approach is particularly useful for seniors who may have sensitive skin or bruising.

It is also important to consider the overall health and well-being of the senior when using acupressure. Some older adults may have medical conditions that require special care or attention. For example, seniors with diabetes may have reduced sensation in their feet, which can make it difficult to apply pressure without causing injury. It is essential to consult with a healthcare provider before using acupressure with seniors who have underlying medical conditions.

In addition to the physical benefits of acupressure, this technique can also have positive psychological effects on seniors. Many older adults experience feelings of isolation and loneliness, particularly if they live alone or have limited social support. Acupressure can help to promote feelings of relaxation and well-being, which can improve overall mood and quality of life.

Acupressure can also be used as a complementary therapy alongside other treatments, such as medication or physical therapy. This approach can help to improve overall health and well-being, and may reduce the need for medication or other invasive treatments.

Addressing Age-Related Issues

Acupressure is a complementary therapy that has been practiced for centuries in traditional Chinese medicine. It involves applying pressure to specific points on the body, known as acupoints, to stimulate the body's natural healing abilities. Acupressure has been shown to be effective for treating a wide range of conditions, and it can also be used to promote overall health and well-being. Below we will explore how acupressure can be used to address age-related issues.

As people age, they often experience a range of physical and mental health issues. These can include chronic pain, arthritis, osteoporosis, insomnia, depression, and anxiety, among others. Acupressure can be an effective way to address these issues, either as a standalone therapy or in combination with other treatments.

One of the benefits of acupressure is that it is a non-invasive therapy that does not involve the use of medication. This makes it a particularly attractive option for older adults who may be taking multiple medications and wish to avoid adding to their medication load. Additionally, acupressure is generally considered safe for older adults, as long as it is performed by a qualified practitioner.

Acupressure can be used to address chronic pain, which is a common issue among older adults. By stimulating specific acupoints, acupressure can help to release tension in the muscles, improve circulation, and reduce inflammation. This can be particularly effective for conditions such as arthritis, which are often associated with chronic pain.

Osteoporosis is another age-related condition that can be addressed with acupressure. By stimulating specific acupoints, acupressure can help to strengthen the bones and reduce the risk of fractures. This can be particularly important for older adults who are at higher risk of falls and fractures.

Insomnia is a common issue among older adults, and acupressure can be an effective way to address this issue. By stimulating specific acupoints, acupressure can help to reduce stress and anxiety, promote relaxation, and improve sleep quality. This can be particularly beneficial for older adults who may be experiencing sleep disturbances due to chronic pain, anxiety, or other health issues.

Depression and anxiety are also common issues among older adults, and acupressure can be an effective way to address these issues. By stimulating specific acupoints, acupressure can help to reduce stress and anxiety, improve mood, and promote a sense of well-being. This can be particularly beneficial for older adults who may be experiencing feelings of isolation or loneliness.

In addition to addressing specific health issues, acupressure can also be used to promote overall health and well-being in older adults. By stimulating specific acupoints, acupressure can help to improve circulation, boost the immune system, and promote relaxation. This can help to reduce the risk of a range of health issues and promote overall vitality and well-being.

When using acupressure with older adults, it is important to take into account any health issues or medical conditions that they may have. For example, acupressure may need to be modified for individuals with cardiovascular issues or blood clotting disorders. Additionally, acupressure should be performed by a qualified practitioner who is familiar with working with older adults and can tailor the therapy to meet their specific needs.

Enhancing Quality of Life

Acupressure is a technique that can help improve the quality of life for people of all ages, including older adults. As we age, our bodies undergo a range of changes that can lead to physical discomfort and decreased mobility. Acupressure can be a valuable tool for addressing these issues and enhancing overall well-being.

One way that acupressure can help older adults is by relieving pain and stiffness in the joints and muscles. As we age, our bodies become less flexible and more prone to inflammation and pain. This can make it difficult to engage in physical activities and may even interfere with daily tasks. Acupressure targets specific points on the body to promote relaxation and release tension, helping to reduce pain and improve mobility.

Another benefit of acupressure for older adults is that it can help improve sleep quality. Sleep disturbances are common among older adults, and can have a negative impact on overall health and well-being. Acupressure can help promote relaxation and reduce stress, making it easier to fall asleep and stay asleep throughout the night.

Acupressure can also be a useful tool for managing age-related conditions such as high blood pressure and arthritis. By targeting specific points on the body, acupressure can help regulate blood flow and reduce inflammation, which may help alleviate symptoms of these conditions.

In addition to physical benefits, acupressure can also be beneficial for mental and emotional health. Older adults may experience increased feelings of anxiety or depression as a result of changes in their lives, such as retirement, loss of loved ones, or health issues. Acupressure can help promote relaxation and reduce stress, which can help improve mood and overall mental well-being.

Adapting acupressure techniques for older adults involves some considerations. One important factor to consider is the comfort and safety of the individual. Older adults may have fragile skin or be more susceptible to injury, so it is important to use gentle pressure and avoid sensitive areas. In addition, some older adults may have underlying health conditions that require modifications to the acupressure techniques used.

Chapter Sixteen

Acupressure for Animals

Acupressure is a traditional healing practice that has been used for centuries to alleviate pain, reduce stress, and promote relaxation. While it is commonly associated with human health, acupressure is also used on animals to promote physical and emotional well-being. This practice is known as animal acupressure and is becoming increasingly popular among pet owners and animal care professionals.

Animal acupressure is a non-invasive therapy that involves applying pressure to specific points on an animal's body. The pressure is applied with the fingers or with specialized tools, such as acupressure balls or pads. The points targeted are the same as those used in human acupressure, and are believed to correspond to specific organs and bodily functions.

The goal of animal acupressure is to balance the animal's energy and promote the natural healing process. This is done by stimulating the flow of Qi, which is the vital life force energy that flows through all living beings. When Qi flows freely, the body is able to maintain optimal health and balance.

Animal acupressure can be used to treat a variety of conditions, both physical and emotional. It is often used to alleviate pain and inflammation, improve circulation, and promote relaxation. It can also be used to treat behavioral issues, such as anxiety and aggression, by promoting a sense of calm and well-being.

Animal acupressure is particularly beneficial for animals who may not be able to tolerate traditional forms of medical treatment, such as medication or surgery. It is also a useful complement to other forms of treatment, such as physical therapy or chiropractic care.

One of the most common uses of animal acupressure is for pain management. It can be used to treat a variety of conditions that cause pain, such as arthritis, hip dysplasia, and spinal injuries. By stimulating specific acupressure points, the body is able to release endorphins, which are natural painkillers. This can provide relief from pain without the need for medication or other invasive treatments.

Another area where animal acupressure is commonly used is in the treatment of anxiety and stress-related disorders. Many animals, particularly dogs and cats, suffer from anxiety and fear-related behaviors. These behaviors can be triggered by a variety of factors, such as loud noises, separation anxiety, or changes in routine. By promoting relaxation and reducing stress levels, animal acupressure can help animals to cope with these triggers and reduce their anxiety.

Animal acupressure can also be used to support the immune system and promote overall health and well-being. By stimulating specific acupressure points, the body is able to release toxins and improve circulation. This can help to boost the immune system and improve overall health.

It is important to note that animal acupressure should only be performed by a trained professional. While it is generally safe, it is important to ensure that the practitioner has experience working with animals and has received proper training in animal acupressure techniques.

In addition, animal acupressure should not be used as a substitute for veterinary care. It is important to consult with a veterinarian before using acupressure or any other alternative therapy on an animal, particularly if the animal has a serious medical condition.

Understanding Animal Meridians

Acupressure is a traditional Chinese healing practice that involves applying pressure to specific points on the body to promote healing, relaxation, and overall well-being. While often associated with human health, acupressure can also be beneficial for animals. In fact, acupressure has been used for centuries in Traditional Chinese Veterinary Medicine (TCVM) to treat a wide range of conditions in both domesticated and wild animals.

To understand how acupressure can benefit animals, it's important to first understand the concept of meridians. In TCVM, meridians are pathways in the body through which energy flows. These meridians correspond to different organs and body systems, and when energy flow is blocked or disrupted, it can lead to illness or other health issues. Acupressure works by stimulating specific points along these meridians to restore the flow of energy and promote healing.

While the basic principles of acupressure are the same for animals and humans, there are some key differences to keep in mind. For example, animals have a different anatomy than humans, so the location of acupressure points will vary depending on the animal species. Additionally, animals may be more sensitive to pressure than humans, so it's important to use a gentle touch and proceed slowly when applying pressure.

Acupressure can be used to treat a wide range of conditions in animals, from musculoskeletal problems to digestive issues and even behavioral problems. Some of the most common uses of acupressure in animals include:

1. Pain relief: Acupressure can be an effective way to relieve pain in animals, particularly those suffering from chronic conditions like arthritis or back pain.

2. Digestive issues: Acupressure can be used to stimulate the digestive system and help alleviate symptoms of constipation, diarrhea, and other gastrointestinal issues.

3. Anxiety and stress: Acupressure can help to calm animals and reduce stress and anxiety, making it useful for animals who are nervous or agitated.

4. Respiratory problems: Acupressure can help to clear blockages in the respiratory system and promote better breathing in animals with respiratory issues.

5. Immune system support: Acupressure can help to boost the immune system and improve overall health in animals.

In addition to its many physical benefits, acupressure can also be a great way to bond with your animal and promote relaxation and well-being. It can be a particularly useful tool for animal caregivers who are looking for natural and non-invasive ways to support their animal's health and wellness.

When working with animals, it's important to approach acupressure with care and caution. If your animal has an underlying health condition or is experiencing a medical emergency, it's always best to seek professional veterinary care. Additionally, it's important to work with a trained acupressure practitioner who is experienced in working with animals and understands their unique needs and sensitivities.

Treating Common Pet Ailments

Acupressure, an ancient healing art, is not just for humans. It can also benefit our furry friends. Acupressure for animals involves the application of pressure to specific points on their body to promote healing, relieve pain, and improve overall well-being. It can be used in conjunction with conventional veterinary care or as a standalone therapy.

To understand how acupressure works on animals, it is important to have a basic understanding of their meridian system. Meridians are energy pathways that run through the body and are connected to organs and bodily functions. Animals have their own meridian system, which is similar to that of humans.

In Traditional Chinese Medicine (TCM), it is believed that when the flow of energy, or Qi, through the meridians is blocked or imbalanced, illness and pain occur. By applying pressure to specific points on the meridians, acupressure can restore balance to the energy flow and promote healing.

Acupressure can be used to treat a wide range of conditions in animals, from chronic pain to behavioral issues. It can also be used as a preventive measure to maintain good health and promote relaxation.

One of the most common conditions that acupressure can help with in animals is arthritis. Arthritis is a degenerative joint disease that affects many older pets. Acupressure can help relieve pain, stiffness, and inflammation associated with arthritis. It can also improve joint mobility and flexibility, making it easier for pets to move around.

Another common condition that acupressure can help with is anxiety. Many pets suffer from anxiety and stress, which can manifest in destructive behavior, excessive barking or meowing, and other unwanted behaviors. Acupressure can help promote relaxation, reduce stress and anxiety, and improve overall emotional well-being.

Acupressure can also be used to treat digestive issues in animals. It can help stimulate digestion, improve appetite, and relieve constipation. This can be particularly beneficial for older pets who may have difficulty digesting food or who suffer from chronic digestive issues.

In addition to these conditions, acupressure can also be used to treat skin and coat issues, respiratory problems, and even cancer. It is a safe and non-invasive therapy that can be used alone or in conjunction with conventional veterinary care.

When performing acupressure on animals, it is important to use gentle techniques and to be aware of any signs of discomfort or pain. Animals may not always be able to communicate their discomfort, so it is important to monitor their response and adjust the pressure accordingly.

Acupressure can be performed by a trained practitioner or by pet owners themselves. There are many resources available for pet owners who wish to learn how to perform acupressure on their own pets. It is important to receive proper training and guidance to ensure that acupressure is performed safely and effectively.

Acupressure for Animal Wellness

Acupressure is a non-invasive technique that can be used to support the health and wellness of animals. Like humans, animals also have energy channels and points that can be stimulated to promote healing and balance in the body. Acupressure is a form of Traditional Chinese Medicine (TCM) that has been used for thousands of years to treat various conditions in both humans and animals.

Acupressure works by applying pressure to specific points along the meridians or energy channels in the body. These points are called acupoints and are located throughout the body. By applying pressure to these points, energy flow is regulated, promoting healing and balance in the body. Acupressure can be used to address a wide range of conditions in animals, including pain, anxiety, digestive issues, and more.

Understanding Animal Meridians

In TCM, the energy channels or meridians in the body are the pathways through which vital energy, known as Qi, flows. Qi travels through these meridians, supplying energy and nourishment to the various organs and tissues of the body. There are twelve primary meridians in the body, each associated with a specific organ system. In addition to the primary meridians, there are also eight extraordinary meridians that are considered to be deeper and more significant than the primary meridians.

In animals, the meridians are similar to those in humans, with some minor differences. For example, in horses, the meridians tend to be longer and wider than in other animals. Understanding the meridian system in animals is essential for acupressure practitioners as they must be able to locate and stimulate the appropriate acupoints for each animal.

Treating Common Pet Ailments

Acupressure can be used to treat a wide range of conditions in animals. Some of the most common conditions that can be addressed with acupressure include pain, anxiety, digestive issues, and respiratory problems.

One of the most common applications of acupressure in animals is for pain management. Acupressure can be used to alleviate pain caused by conditions such as arthritis, hip dysplasia, and back pain. By stimulating specific acupoints, acupressure can help to reduce inflammation, increase blood flow, and release endorphins, which are natural painkillers produced by the body.

Acupressure can also be used to address anxiety and behavioral issues in animals. By stimulating specific acupoints, acupressure can help to calm the nervous system, reduce stress, and promote relaxation. This can be particularly beneficial for animals that suffer from separation anxiety, fear of loud noises, or other phobias.

Digestive issues are another common condition that can be addressed with acupressure. Acupressure can help to regulate digestion and reduce symptoms such as vomiting, diarrhea, and constipation. By stimulating specific acupoints, acupressure can help to regulate the digestive system, increase appetite, and improve nutrient absorption.

Respiratory problems are also a common condition that can be addressed with acupressure. Acupressure can help to clear congestion, reduce inflammation, and promote healing in the respiratory system. This can be particularly beneficial for animals that suffer from conditions such as asthma, bronchitis, or allergies.

Acupressure for Animal Wellness

In addition to addressing specific conditions, acupressure can also be used to promote overall wellness in animals. Regular acupressure sessions can help to maintain optimal health and prevent illness. Acupressure can also be used to improve immune function, increase energy, and promote mental and emotional balance.

Acupressure can be particularly beneficial for animals that are recovering from illness or injury. By stimulating specific acup

Chapter Seventeen

Acupressure for Beauty and Skincare

Acupressure is an ancient healing technique that involves the application of pressure to specific points on the body to improve physical, mental, and emotional health. Over the years, acupressure has been used for various purposes, including beauty and skincare. This chapter explores the concept of acupressure for beauty and skincare, the science behind it, and the benefits it offers.

Acupressure for beauty and skincare involves the use of specific acupoints on the face and body to promote healthy skin and enhance one's appearance. According to Traditional Chinese Medicine (TCM), the face has several meridians that correspond to various organs in the body. By applying pressure to specific points on the face, acupressure can stimulate blood circulation and energy flow, which promotes skin health.

The science behind acupressure lies in the belief that the human body has a natural healing mechanism that can be activated by stimulating specific points on the body. In TCM, these points are referred to as acupoints, and they are believed to be connected by a network of channels or meridians that run throughout the body. By stimulating these points, acupressure can help the body restore balance and promote healing.

Acupressure for beauty and skincare involves the use of specific acupoints on the face, neck, and body to address various skin issues. For example, acupressure can help improve the appearance of fine lines, wrinkles, and dark circles around the eyes. It can also help reduce inflammation and redness, promote collagen production, and improve skin tone and texture.

One of the primary benefits of acupressure for beauty and skincare is that it is a natural and non-invasive technique that does not involve the use of any chemicals or harsh treatments. This makes it an excellent alternative to traditional skincare treatments that can be expensive and may have adverse side effects. Acupressure is also a holistic approach to skincare that considers the body and mind as a whole, rather than just addressing specific symptoms.

Acupressure for beauty and skincare can also be used in conjunction with other natural skincare practices, such as facial massage, meditation, and yoga, to enhance their effectiveness. By promoting relaxation and reducing stress, acupressure can help improve overall skin health and radiance.

Some of the most popular acupoints used in acupressure for beauty and skincare include the forehead point, located between the eyebrows, which is said to promote relaxation and reduce tension; the temple point, located at the temples, which can help relieve headaches and eye strain; and the jaw point, located at the jawline, which can help reduce puffiness and promote lymphatic drainage.

Other acupoints used in acupressure for beauty and skincare include the neck point, located at the base of the neck, which can help reduce tension and promote blood flow to the face; the shoulder point, located at the top of the shoulders, which can help relieve stress and tension; and the ear points, which can help reduce inflammation and promote relaxation.

Acupressure Facelift Techniques

Acupressure is a form of traditional Chinese medicine that involves applying pressure to specific points on the body. In recent years, acupressure has gained popularity in the beauty and skincare industry for its purported ability to provide a natural facelift. Acupressure facelift techniques are becoming increasingly popular as a non-invasive alternative to traditional facelift surgery. Below we will explore the benefits of acupressure facelift techniques and how they work.

Acupressure facelift techniques are based on the principles of traditional Chinese medicine. According to this ancient practice, energy flows through the body along channels known as meridians. By applying pressure to specific points on these meridians, the flow of energy can be restored, promoting health and wellness.

In the context of skincare, acupressure facelift techniques are believed to work by stimulating the production of collagen and elastin, two proteins that are essential for healthy skin. Collagen and elastin provide structure and elasticity to the skin, keeping it firm and smooth. As we age, the production of these proteins decreases, leading to wrinkles and sagging skin.

Acupressure facelift techniques involve applying pressure to specific points on the face, neck, and shoulders. These points correspond to different meridians in the body and are believed to promote the flow of energy and stimulate the production of collagen and elastin.

One popular acupressure facelift technique is known as the "facial glow" or "facial rejuvenation" technique. This technique involves applying gentle pressure to specific points on the face, such as the temples, cheeks, and jawline. The pressure is applied in a circular motion, with the fingers moving in a clockwise direction. This technique is believed to promote blood flow and stimulate the production of collagen and elastin, leading to a more youthful, glowing complexion.

Another popular acupressure facelift technique is known as the "facial cupping" technique. This technique involves using small suction cups to massage the face and neck. The cups are placed on specific points on the face and moved in a gentle, circular motion. This technique is believed to promote lymphatic drainage and increase blood flow, leading to a brighter, more radiant complexion.

Acupressure facelift techniques are also believed to have a relaxing effect on the body and mind. The application of pressure to specific points on the body is believed to release tension and promote relaxation. This can help to reduce stress and anxiety, which can have a positive impact on overall health and well-being.

While acupressure facelift techniques are generally considered safe, it is important to note that they should not be used as a replacement for traditional medical treatments. If you have any underlying health conditions, it is important to speak with your healthcare provider before attempting any acupressure techniques.

In addition, it is important to seek out a qualified and experienced acupressure practitioner if you are interested in pursuing acupressure facelift techniques. A trained practitioner can help you identify the appropriate pressure points and techniques for your specific needs, ensuring that you get the best results possible.

Pressure Points for Skin Health

Acupressure is an ancient healing technique that has been used for centuries to treat various health conditions. This technique involves the application of pressure to specific points on the body, known as acupoints, to stimulate the body's natural healing response. While acupressure is commonly known for its ability to relieve pain, it can also be beneficial for improving skin health.

Acupressure works by stimulating the body's meridian system, a network of pathways that carry vital energy or "Qi" throughout the body. These pathways correspond to different organs and systems in the body, and when they become blocked or imbalanced, it can lead to various health problems, including skin issues.

There are several acupressure points that can help improve skin health, including:

LI4 (Hegu) - This point is located on the back of the hand between the thumb and index finger. It is believed to help promote overall skin health and relieve skin conditions such as acne, eczema, and rashes.

ST36 (Zusanli) - This point is located on the lower leg, about four finger widths below the knee. It is believed to help promote skin elasticity and improve complexion.

GV14 (Dazhui) - This point is located at the base of the neck, in the center of the spine. It is believed to help promote skin health and relieve skin conditions such as acne and psoriasis.

LI11 (Quchi) - This point is located on the outer side of the elbow. It is believed to help detoxify the skin and promote skin health.

SP6 (Sanyinjiao) - This point is located on the inner side of the leg, about four finger widths above the ankle. It is believed to help regulate hormones and improve skin conditions such as acne and eczema.

In addition to stimulating these acupressure points, there are also several techniques that can be used to improve skin health. One of these techniques is known as gua sha, which involves using a small tool to scrape the skin in a specific pattern. This technique can help stimulate blood flow, reduce inflammation, and promote lymphatic drainage, all of which can improve skin health.

Another technique that can be used is facial acupressure massage. This involves applying gentle pressure to specific points on the face to improve circulation and promote lymphatic drainage. This technique can help reduce puffiness, improve skin tone, and reduce the appearance of fine lines and wrinkles.

It's important to note that while acupressure can be beneficial for improving skin health, it should not be used as a substitute for professional medical advice. If you have a skin condition that is causing discomfort or is not improving with self-care, it's important to consult with a healthcare professional for proper diagnosis and treatment.

In addition to acupressure, there are several other lifestyle factors that can help improve skin health, including maintaining a healthy diet, staying hydrated, getting enough sleep, and avoiding smoking and excessive alcohol consumption. By incorporating these practices into your daily routine and working with a healthcare professional when needed, you can help promote healthy, vibrant skin.

Combining Acupressure with Skincare Regimens

Acupressure is an ancient healing technique that has been used for thousands of years to treat a variety of physical and mental conditions. In recent years, acupressure has gained popularity in the beauty and skincare industry as a natural and non-invasive alternative to traditional cosmetic procedures. Acupressure can be easily integrated into a skincare routine and can provide numerous benefits, including improved circulation, enhanced skin tone, and reduced signs of aging. Below we will explore the benefits of combining acupressure with skincare regimens.

Acupressure works by stimulating specific pressure points on the body that correspond to different organs and systems. These pressure points can be found throughout the body, including on the face and scalp. When these pressure points are stimulated, it can increase blood flow and energy flow, which can help to improve the overall health and appearance of the skin.

One of the most popular acupressure techniques for skincare is the acupressure facelift. This technique involves using the fingers to massage specific pressure points on the face and neck to help tighten and tone the skin. The acupressure facelift can help to reduce the appearance of wrinkles and fine lines, as well as improve the overall texture and tone of the skin.

Another popular acupressure technique for skincare is the use of jade rollers. Jade rollers are small, handheld devices that are made from jade or other precious stones. They are designed to be rolled over the face and neck, and can help to improve circulation, reduce puffiness, and promote lymphatic drainage. Jade rollers are often used in combination with facial oils or serums to help improve the absorption of these products into the skin.

In addition to the acupressure facelift and jade rollers, there are many other acupressure techniques that can be used to promote healthy skin. For example, stimulating the pressure points on the ears can help to improve circulation to the face and reduce the appearance of dark circles and puffiness under the eyes. Massaging the pressure points on the scalp can also help to promote healthy hair growth and improve the overall health of the scalp.

When combining acupressure with a skincare regimen, it is important to use high-quality skincare products that are free from harmful chemicals and toxins. This can help to ensure that the skin is receiving the nutrients and hydration it needs to stay healthy and vibrant. Additionally, it is important to maintain a healthy diet and lifestyle, as this can also have a significant impact on the health and appearance of the skin.

It is also important to note that acupressure should not be used as a substitute for medical treatment. While acupressure can be a beneficial addition to a skincare regimen, it is important to seek professional medical advice for any skin conditions or concerns.

Chapter Eighteen

Acupressure for Weight Management

Acupressure is an alternative therapy that has gained popularity for its effectiveness in managing various health conditions, including weight management. It is based on the principle that applying pressure to specific points on the body can stimulate the body's natural healing mechanisms and restore balance. Acupressure can help with weight management by regulating appetite, reducing stress, and improving digestion.

One of the most effective ways acupressure can help with weight management is by regulating appetite. The practice involves applying pressure to specific points on the body, which can help to control hunger and reduce cravings. Acupressure targets the acupoints that are associated with the digestive system and can help to increase the body's metabolism, thereby promoting weight loss.

One of the acupoints that can help with appetite control is the ear point. The ear point is located on the outer ear and can be stimulated by applying gentle pressure with the fingers or using ear seeds. Ear seeds are small seeds that are placed on the ear and are left there for a few days. The seeds can help to stimulate the ear point, which can reduce cravings and help to control hunger.

Another way that acupressure can help with weight management is by reducing stress. Stress can lead to emotional eating and can make it difficult to stick to a healthy diet. Acupressure can help to reduce stress by stimulating the body's natural relaxation response. By applying pressure to specific acupoints, the body can release tension and promote feelings of calm and relaxation. This can help to reduce stress and improve overall well-being, which can support healthy eating habits and weight management.

One of the most effective acupoints for reducing stress is the Heart 7 point. The Heart 7 point is located on the inner wrist and can be stimulated by applying gentle pressure with the fingers. The Heart 7 point can help to calm the mind and promote relaxation, which can reduce stress and improve mood. By reducing stress, acupressure can help to prevent emotional eating and support healthy weight management.

Acupressure can also help to improve digestion, which can support weight management. Poor digestion can lead to bloating, constipation, and other digestive issues that can make it difficult to lose weight. Acupressure can help to improve digestion by stimulating the digestive system and promoting healthy gut function.

One of the most effective acupoints for improving digestion is the Stomach 36 point. The Stomach 36 point is located on the lower leg and can be stimulated by applying pressure with the fingers. This acupoint can help to improve digestion by promoting the production of digestive enzymes and supporting healthy gut function. By improving digestion, acupressure can help to support weight management and improve overall health.

Pressure Points for Appetite Control

Acupressure is an ancient healing art that involves applying pressure to specific points on the body to promote health and wellness. One area where acupressure is gaining popularity is in weight management. By targeting specific pressure points, acupressure can help reduce appetite and cravings, boost metabolism, and improve digestion. Below we will explore the pressure points that are effective for appetite control and weight management.

The first pressure point that is commonly used for appetite control is the ear point. The ear has several acupressure points that are connected to various organs in the body, including the stomach and spleen. By stimulating these points, you can reduce hunger and cravings, as well as improve digestion. The most effective point for appetite control is the hunger point, which is located in the innermost part of the ear. To activate this point, use your thumb and index finger to apply gentle pressure to the ear lobe and move upwards towards the top of the ear.

Another pressure point that is effective for weight management is the Third Eye point. This point is located between the eyebrows and is connected to the pituitary gland, which plays a key role in regulating appetite and metabolism. By stimulating this point, you can boost your metabolism and reduce cravings. To activate this point, use your index finger to apply gentle pressure to the Third Eye point and hold for several seconds.

The Abdomen point is another effective pressure point for weight management. This point is located three finger widths below the belly button and is connected to the digestive system. By stimulating this point, you can improve digestion and reduce bloating, which can help you feel fuller for longer. To activate this point, use your index and middle fingers to apply gentle pressure to the Abdomen point and hold for several seconds.

The Four Gates point is also effective for appetite control and weight management. This point is located on the back of the hand, between the index finger and thumb. By stimulating this point, you can reduce stress and anxiety, which can often trigger overeating. To activate this point, use your thumb and index finger to apply gentle pressure to the Four Gates point and hold for several seconds.

The Stomach point is another effective pressure point for appetite control. This point is located two finger widths below the kneecap, on the outer edge of the shinbone. By stimulating this point, you can reduce cravings and improve digestion. To activate this point, use your index and middle fingers to apply gentle pressure to the Stomach point and hold for several seconds.

In addition to these pressure points, there are also several acupressure techniques that can be used to promote weight management. One of these techniques is the stomach massage, which involves gently massaging the stomach area in a clockwise direction. This helps to stimulate digestion and reduce bloating, which can help you feel fuller for longer.

Another acupressure technique that is effective for weight management is the ear massage. This involves gently massaging the ear lobe and surrounding areas to stimulate the hunger point and reduce cravings. This technique can be done throughout the day, as needed.

It is important to note that acupressure should not be used as a standalone weight management technique. It should be used in combination with a healthy diet and regular exercise. Acupressure can help reduce appetite and cravings, boost metabolism, and improve digestion, but it is not a magic solution for weight loss.

Supporting Digestion and Metabolism

Acupressure, a traditional Chinese healing method, is gaining popularity as a natural way to support digestion and metabolism. The practice involves applying pressure to specific points on the body known as acupoints, which correspond to the meridian channels of energy flow in the body. Acupressure stimulates the body's natural healing abilities, helping to regulate digestion and improve metabolism.

The digestive system is responsible for breaking down food into nutrients and eliminating waste. It is a complex process that involves many organs, including the stomach, pancreas, liver, and intestines. Digestive issues such as bloating, constipation, and acid reflux can occur when the digestive system is not functioning properly. Acupressure can help to alleviate these symptoms by stimulating digestion and improving the flow of energy through the digestive organs.

One of the most effective acupressure points for supporting digestion is the Stomach 36 (ST36) point. This point is located on the leg, about four finger widths below the knee and one finger width to the outside of the shin bone. Stimulating this point helps to regulate digestion, alleviate bloating and constipation, and reduce inflammation in the digestive system. To stimulate the ST36 point, apply firm pressure with the fingertips and massage in a circular motion for several minutes.

Another acupressure point that can help to support digestion is the Pericardium 6 (PC6) point. This point is located on the inside of the wrist, about three finger widths up from the wrist crease. Stimulating this point can alleviate nausea, vomiting, and heartburn. To stimulate the PC6 point, apply firm pressure with the fingertips and massage in a circular motion for several minutes.

Acupressure can also be used to support metabolism, which is the process by which the body converts food into energy. A sluggish metabolism can lead to weight gain and other health issues. The Triple Burner 23 (TB23) point is one of the most effective acupressure points for supporting metabolism. This point is located on the face, in the hollows between the eyebrows and the bridge of the nose. Stimulating this point can help to boost metabolism, improve digestion, and reduce cravings. To stimulate the TB23 point, apply firm pressure with the fingertips and massage in a circular motion for several minutes.

In addition to acupressure, there are several other natural ways to support digestion and metabolism. Eating a healthy diet that is rich in fiber, lean protein, and healthy fats can help to support digestion and boost metabolism. Drinking plenty of water can also help to flush out toxins and support digestion.

Regular exercise is another key factor in supporting metabolism. Exercise helps to build muscle mass, which in turn helps to increase metabolism. It also helps to reduce stress, which can interfere with digestion and metabolism.

Stress reduction techniques such as meditation, deep breathing, and yoga can also be beneficial for supporting digestion and metabolism. Stress can interfere with the body's natural healing abilities, leading to digestive issues and a sluggish metabolism. By reducing stress, the body is better able to regulate digestion and boost metabolism.

Combining Acupressure with a Healthy Lifestyle

Acupressure is a natural and non-invasive healing modality that involves the application of pressure on specific points on the body. This ancient healing practice has been used for centuries to alleviate various health problems, including chronic pain, anxiety, and digestive issues. Acupressure can also be an effective tool to support a healthy lifestyle when combined with a nutritious diet and regular exercise. Below we will explore the benefits of combining acupressure with a healthy lifestyle and provide some tips on how to integrate this practice into your daily routine.

One of the main benefits of acupressure is that it can help regulate the body's systems, including the digestive and metabolic systems. By applying pressure on specific points on the body, acupressure can stimulate the digestive organs, helping to improve digestion and nutrient absorption.

This can lead to better energy levels and an overall sense of well-being. Acupressure can also help regulate the metabolism, which can aid in weight loss or weight management.

To support a healthy lifestyle, it is important to incorporate a well-balanced diet and regular exercise into your routine. A healthy diet should consist of whole, nutrient-dense foods, such as fruits, vegetables, lean proteins, and whole grains. Regular exercise can help maintain a healthy weight, improve cardiovascular health, and increase overall strength and endurance. However, these lifestyle changes can sometimes be challenging to incorporate and maintain. This is where acupressure can be a useful tool.

Acupressure can be used to support healthy digestion by targeting specific points on the body. One of these points is known as Stomach 36, which is located on the lower leg. By applying pressure on this point, it can help alleviate digestive issues, such as bloating, constipation, and indigestion. To apply pressure on this point, use your fingers to apply a firm pressure for about 30 seconds, and repeat several times a day.

Another point that can support digestion and metabolism is known as Spleen 6, located on the inner ankle. This point can help regulate the digestive system and improve blood flow to the digestive organs. To apply pressure on this point, use your fingers to apply a firm pressure for about 30 seconds, and repeat several times a day.

Acupressure can also help support a healthy immune system, which is essential for overall well-being. One of the points that can help support the immune system is known as Large Intestine 4, located on the hand. By applying pressure on this point, it can help alleviate cold and flu symptoms and improve overall immunity. To apply pressure on this point, use your fingers to apply a firm pressure for about 30 seconds, and repeat several times a day.

To incorporate acupressure into your daily routine, try setting aside a few minutes each day to apply pressure on specific points on the body. This can be done while watching TV, during a break at work, or before going to bed. By incorporating acupressure into your daily routine, it can help alleviate stress and tension, improve overall health and well-being, and support a healthy lifestyle.

In addition to acupressure, other holistic practices can also support a healthy lifestyle. Meditation, yoga, and tai chi are all practices that can help reduce stress, improve flexibility and balance, and promote overall health and well-being. These practices can be incorporated into your daily routine alongside acupressure to create a well-rounded approach to a healthy lifestyle.

Chapter Nineteen

Acupressure for Travel and Jet Lag

Acupressure, an ancient healing technique that involves applying pressure to specific points on the body, has been shown to be effective in treating a variety of conditions. One of these conditions is travel-related issues such as jet lag, motion sickness, and stress. Below we will explore how acupressure can help alleviate the symptoms of travel and jet lag and how it can be incorporated into a traveler's routine.

Jet lag is a common condition that affects people who travel across multiple time zones. It is caused by a disruption in the body's natural sleep-wake cycle, which can result in fatigue, insomnia, and other symptoms. Acupressure can help alleviate these symptoms by stimulating the body's natural healing mechanisms.

One of the acupressure points that can help with jet lag is the Pericardium 6 (PC6) point. This point is located on the inside of the wrist, about two finger widths from the crease where the hand meets the wrist. Stimulating this point can help alleviate nausea, headaches, and other symptoms associated with jet lag.

Another acupressure point that can help with jet lag is the Bladder 62 (BL62) point. This point is located on the outside of the ankle, just below the ankle bone. Stimulating this point can help with insomnia, fatigue, and other symptoms associated with jet lag.

In addition to these specific acupressure points, there are also general techniques that can help alleviate travel-related issues. One technique is to apply pressure to the base of the skull, which can help alleviate tension headaches and neck pain. Another technique is to massage the feet, which can help improve circulation and reduce swelling.

Acupressure can also be effective in treating motion sickness, which is a common issue for travelers. The Pericardium 6 (PC6) point, which was mentioned earlier, is effective in treating nausea associated with motion sickness. Another acupressure point that can help with motion sickness is the Stomach 36 (ST36) point. This point is located on the leg, about four finger widths below the kneecap. Stimulating this point can help alleviate nausea and vomiting.

In addition to these specific acupressure points, there are also general techniques that can help alleviate motion sickness. One technique is to apply pressure to the inner wrist, between the tendons. Another technique is to massage the temples, which can help alleviate headaches and dizziness.

Acupressure can also be effective in reducing stress and anxiety associated with travel. The Governing Vessel 24.5 (GV24.5) point, also known as the "Third Eye" point, is an acupressure point that can help alleviate stress and anxiety. This point is located between the eyebrows, in the center of the forehead. Stimulating this point can help calm the mind and reduce anxiety.

Another acupressure point that can help with stress and anxiety is the Heart 7 (HT7) point. This point is located on the inside of the wrist, just above the crease where the hand meets the wrist. Stimulating this point can help alleviate anxiety and promote relaxation.

In addition to these specific acupressure points, there are also general techniques that can help alleviate stress and anxiety. One technique is to focus on deep breathing, which can help calm the mind and reduce stress. Another technique is to practice mindfulness, which involves being fully present in the moment and focusing on the present experience.

Pressure Points for Motion Sickness

Acupressure is a technique that has been used for centuries to help relieve a variety of ailments, including motion sickness. Motion sickness can be caused by many factors, including travel on a boat, car, or plane, and can be a very unpleasant experience. However, acupressure can be an effective way to manage motion sickness symptoms without the use of medications or other interventions. Below we will explore the pressure points that are most effective for managing motion sickness and how to properly apply acupressure for best results.

Motion sickness is a common condition that affects many people when they travel. Symptoms of motion sickness can include nausea, vomiting, dizziness, and sweating. These symptoms can be very uncomfortable and can even lead to dehydration if not managed properly. While there are medications available to manage motion sickness, many people prefer natural remedies like acupressure to avoid side effects and potential interactions with other medications.

There are several pressure points that are effective for managing motion sickness symptoms. The first point is located on the wrist and is called the Nei Guan or P6 point. This point is located between the tendons on the inside of the wrist and is easy to locate by placing three fingers below the wrist crease. Applying pressure to this point for a few minutes can help relieve nausea and vomiting.

The second point is located on the leg and is called the Zu San Li point. This point is located four finger-widths below the kneecap on the outside of the leg. Applying pressure to this point can help relieve nausea, vomiting, and dizziness.

The third point is located on the ear and is called the Shen Men or Heavenly Gate point. This point is located in the center of the ear, at the top of the triangular fossa. Applying pressure to this point can help relieve nausea, vomiting, and dizziness.

To apply acupressure to these points, start by finding a comfortable position. You can either sit or stand, but make sure you are relaxed and not tense. Begin by applying firm pressure to the selected point using your thumb or fingers. Apply pressure for a few minutes or until you feel relief from your symptoms. You can also use circular motions or massage the point to help stimulate the pressure point.

In addition to acupressure, there are other lifestyle changes that can help manage motion sickness symptoms. These include eating a light meal before traveling, avoiding strong odors or foods that trigger nausea, staying hydrated, and taking frequent breaks to get fresh air and stretch your legs.

It is important to note that while acupressure can be an effective way to manage motion sickness, it may not work for everyone. It is always a good idea to consult with a healthcare professional before trying any new treatment or remedy.

Reducing Jet Lag Symptoms

Jet lag is a common condition that affects travelers who cross multiple time zones, causing symptoms such as fatigue, sleep disturbances, and digestive problems. While there are several ways to manage jet lag, such as adjusting sleep schedules, staying hydrated, and avoiding alcohol and caffeine, acupressure is a natural and effective technique that can help reduce the symptoms of jet lag. Below we will discuss acupressure techniques that can be used to reduce the symptoms of jet lag and help travelers adjust to new time zones.

Acupressure is a traditional Chinese medicine technique that involves applying pressure to specific points on the body to stimulate energy flow and promote healing. According to traditional Chinese medicine, acupressure works by activating the body's natural healing mechanisms and balancing the flow of energy, or "Qi," through the body's meridians. By applying pressure to specific points on the body, acupressure can help relieve pain, reduce stress, and improve overall health and well-being.

When it comes to managing jet lag, acupressure can be a helpful tool in reducing symptoms and promoting relaxation. The following are some acupressure points that can be targeted to help reduce jet lag symptoms:

The Pericardium 6 (P6) point, also known as the Nei Guan point, is located on the inside of the wrist, about two finger-widths below the crease of the wrist. This point is commonly used to relieve nausea and promote relaxation.

The Liver 3 (LR3) point is located on the top of the foot, between the big toe and the second toe. This point is commonly used to relieve stress and promote relaxation.

The Stomach 36 (ST36) point is located on the lower leg, about four finger-widths below the knee and one finger-width to the outside of the shinbone. This point is commonly used to improve digestion and promote overall health.

The Bladder 62 (BL62) point is located on the ankle, just behind the ankle bone. This point is commonly used to relieve stress and promote relaxation.

By targeting these specific acupressure points, travelers can help alleviate symptoms of jet lag and promote relaxation and well-being.

In addition to targeting specific acupressure points, there are also some general acupressure techniques that can be used to help reduce the symptoms of jet lag. One technique involves placing the hands over the eyes and applying gentle pressure for several minutes. This can help reduce eye strain and promote relaxation. Another technique involves placing the hands on the back of the neck and applying gentle pressure for several minutes. This can help relieve tension and promote relaxation in the neck and shoulders.

While acupressure can be a helpful tool in managing jet lag, it is important to note that it should not be used as a substitute for medical treatment. If you are experiencing severe or persistent symptoms of jet lag, it is important to seek medical attention.

In addition to using acupressure techniques, there are several other ways to manage jet lag and promote healthy sleep habits. These include:

1. Adjusting sleep schedules: In the days leading up to travel, gradually adjust sleep schedules to match the time zone of the destination. This can help the body adjust more easily to the new time zone.

2. Staying hydrated: Drink plenty of water and avoid alcohol and caffeine, which can dehydrate the body and disrupt sleep.

3. Eating healthy: Stick to a healthy diet and avoid heavy, greasy foods that can disrupt digestion and sleep.

4. Exercising: Engage in regular physical activity to promote overall health and well-being.

On-the-Go Acupressure Techniques

On-the-go acupressure techniques are simple and effective ways to reduce stress and promote relaxation while on the move. Whether you are commuting to work, traveling, or simply on a busy schedule, these techniques can help you find relief from tension and discomfort.

Acupressure is a form of alternative therapy that involves applying pressure to specific points on the body. These points, also known as acupoints, are believed to be connected to the body's energy channels or meridians, and stimulating them can help restore balance and promote healing.

One of the benefits of acupressure is that it can be done anywhere, at any time, without the need for any special equipment. Here are some on-the-go acupressure techniques that you can try:

1. Ear massage: The ears contain several acupoints that are believed to promote relaxation and reduce stress. To stimulate these points, gently massage the entire surface of your ears using your fingertips. Start at the top of your ears and work your way down to the lobes, applying a firm but gentle pressure.

2. Scalp massage: Massaging the scalp can help relieve tension and promote relaxation. Use your fingertips to gently rub your scalp in circular motions, focusing on the areas around your temples and the back of your head.

3. Hand acupressure: The hands contain several acupoints that are believed to be connected to different parts of the body. To stimulate these points, use your thumb and index finger to gently pinch the webbing between your fingers. You can also massage the area between your thumb and index finger using circular motions.

4. Foot acupressure: The feet contain numerous acupoints that are believed to promote relaxation and relieve tension throughout the body. To stimulate these points, use your thumb to apply pressure to the center of your foot, just below the ball of your foot. You can also use your fingertips to massage the entire surface of your foot, focusing on the areas around the toes and the heel.

5. Neck and shoulder stretch: The neck and shoulders are common areas where tension and discomfort can build up. To relieve tension in these areas, stretch your neck by gently tilting your head to one side and holding for a few seconds before repeating on the other side. You can also do shoulder rolls by lifting your shoulders up towards your ears, then rolling them back and down in a circular motion.

It's important to note that while acupressure is generally safe, there are some precautions you should take when practicing it on-the-go. Be sure to avoid applying pressure to any areas that are bruised or injured, and stop immediately if you experience any pain or discomfort. Additionally, if you have any pre-existing medical conditions, be sure to talk to your healthcare provider before practicing acupressure.

Chapter Twenty

Acupressure and Traditional Chinese Medicine

Acupressure is an ancient healing art that originated in China thousands of years ago. It is based on the principles of Traditional Chinese Medicine (TCM), which views the body as a complex network of energy channels, or meridians, through which life force energy, or Qi, flows. Acupressure involves applying pressure to specific points on these meridians to stimulate the flow of Qi and promote healing.

TCM is a holistic approach to healthcare that recognizes the interconnectedness of mind, body, and spirit. It is based on the concept of Yin and Yang, the two opposing but complementary forces that exist in all things. Health is seen as a state of balance between these forces, and illness is seen as an imbalance or blockage in the flow of Qi. Acupressure is one of the many therapies used in TCM to restore balance and promote wellness.

There are over 360 acupressure points on the body, each with its unique function and healing properties. The location of these points is determined by the meridians they are associated with, and each meridian is connected to specific organs and body systems. For example, the Lung meridian runs through the arms and is associated with the respiratory system, while the Stomach meridian runs through the abdomen and is associated with digestion.

Acupressure points can be stimulated using finger pressure, massage, or other techniques such as moxibustion, which involves burning the herb mugwort on or near the point to create heat and stimulate the flow of Qi. Acupressure can be used to treat a wide range of physical, emotional, and mental health conditions, including pain, anxiety, depression, insomnia, digestive issues, and menstrual disorders, among others.

In TCM, acupressure is often used in combination with other therapies such as acupuncture, herbal medicine, and dietary therapy. Acupuncture involves inserting thin needles into specific points on the body to stimulate the flow of Qi, while herbal medicine uses natural plant-based remedies to promote healing. Dietary therapy involves using food as medicine to support overall health and balance.

One of the main benefits of acupressure and TCM is that they are a safe and natural approach to healthcare. Unlike many modern Western medical interventions, which often involve the use of drugs or surgery, acupressure works with the body's natural healing processes to promote balance and wellness. This makes it a popular choice for people who prefer a more holistic and gentle approach to healthcare.

Another benefit of acupressure is that it can be easily integrated into daily life. Many acupressure points can be stimulated using simple self-massage techniques, making it a convenient and cost-effective way to promote health and wellbeing. For example, massaging the Stomach 36 point, which is located on the lower leg, can help improve digestion and boost energy levels.

While acupressure is generally safe and well-tolerated, there are some precautions that should be taken. It is important to avoid stimulating certain points during pregnancy, as they can cause contractions and potentially harm the developing fetus. People with certain medical conditions, such as cancer or bleeding disorders, should also avoid acupressure or seek guidance from a qualified healthcare practitioner.

Understanding TCM Concepts

Traditional Chinese Medicine (TCM) is a holistic healthcare system that dates back over 2000 years. It includes various treatment modalities such as acupuncture, herbal medicine, and acupressure, and it is still widely practiced today. TCM is based on the concept that the human body is a microcosm of the larger universe and is subject to the same natural laws. The basic tenets of TCM are rooted in the principles of yin and yang and the five elements.

Yin and yang are the two opposing yet complementary forces that exist in the universe. Yin is associated with cold, darkness, and female energy, while yang is associated with warmth, light, and male energy. According to TCM, the balance of these two forces is crucial for health and well-being.

The five elements, also known as the five phases, are wood, fire, earth, metal, and water. Each element is associated with specific organs, emotions, and qualities. Wood is associated with the liver and gallbladder and represents growth and creativity. Fire is associated with the heart and small intestine and represents joy and passion. Earth is associated with the spleen and stomach and represents nurturing and stability. Metal is associated with the lungs and large intestine and represents clarity and precision. Water is associated with the kidneys and bladder and represents wisdom and adaptability.

TCM also recognizes the existence of Qi, the vital energy that flows through the body along specific pathways called meridians. Qi is said to govern the body's functions and maintain health and well-being. The meridians are like a network of highways that connect different parts of the body and allow the flow of Qi. The meridians are also associated with specific organs and emotions.

Acupressure is one of the TCM modalities that utilize the concept of meridians and Qi. It involves the application of pressure on specific acupoints along the meridians to stimulate the flow of Qi and promote healing. Acupressure can be performed using fingers, hands, elbows, or specialized tools.

In TCM, acupressure is used to treat a wide range of health conditions, including chronic pain, stress, anxiety, digestive problems, and respiratory issues. Acupressure is also used for preventive care and to maintain overall health and well-being.

One of the key benefits of acupressure is that it is a non-invasive and drug-free therapy. Unlike medications or surgeries that can have side effects or complications, acupressure is generally considered safe and well-tolerated. It is also a cost-effective treatment option compared to other healthcare modalities.

Acupressure is often used in conjunction with other TCM modalities, such as herbal medicine and acupuncture, to enhance its effectiveness. For example, acupressure can be used to alleviate pain and discomfort, while herbal medicine can be used to support the body's natural healing process. Acupuncture can also be used to stimulate the flow of Qi and address deeper imbalances in the body.

Combining Acupressure with Herbal Remedies

Acupressure is an ancient healing art that has been practiced for thousands of years. It involves applying pressure to specific points on the body to relieve pain and promote healing. While acupressure can be effective on its own, combining it with herbal remedies can enhance its therapeutic benefits. Below we will discuss the benefits of combining acupressure with herbal remedies and how this approach can be used to promote health and well-being.

Herbal remedies have been used for centuries to treat a wide range of health conditions. Many herbs have anti-inflammatory, analgesic, and antimicrobial properties, making them effective for treating conditions such as arthritis, headaches, and infections. When combined with acupressure, herbal remedies can enhance the healing benefits of this therapy.

One of the ways in which herbal remedies can be used with acupressure is through the use of herbal poultices. A poultice is a mixture of herbs that is applied directly to the skin. When combined with acupressure, the poultice can be applied to specific acupressure points to enhance the healing benefits of the therapy. For example, a poultice made with ginger and turmeric can be applied to the stomach and spleen meridians to relieve digestive problems.

Another way in which herbal remedies can be used with acupressure is through the use of herbal teas. Herbal teas can be used to stimulate the body's natural healing mechanisms and promote relaxation. When combined with acupressure, herbal teas can help to relieve stress and tension, which can contribute to many health conditions.

Herbs such as chamomile, lavender, and passionflower are known for their calming and relaxing properties. When combined with acupressure, these herbs can help to relieve anxiety and promote relaxation. For example, chamomile tea can be consumed before an acupressure session to help the patient relax and get the most benefit from the therapy.

In addition to poultices and teas, herbal remedies can also be used in combination with acupressure through the use of herbal supplements. Herbal supplements can be used to address specific health conditions and can be tailored to the individual needs of the patient. For example, a patient with arthritis may benefit from taking an herbal supplement that contains turmeric and ginger, while a patient with a respiratory infection may benefit from taking an herbal supplement that contains echinacea and goldenseal.

When using herbal supplements with acupressure, it is important to work with a qualified healthcare practitioner who can help to determine the best course of treatment. A practitioner who is knowledgeable in both acupressure and herbal medicine can create a personalized treatment plan that addresses the patient's individual needs and goals.

Incorporating TCM Principles into Your Practice

Acupressure is an ancient healing art that has been used in Traditional Chinese Medicine (TCM) for thousands of years. TCM is a holistic approach to health that aims to balance the body, mind, and spirit by considering the whole person and their environment. TCM includes various modalities such as acupuncture, herbal medicine, cupping, and gua sha. Acupressure is one of the essential tools in TCM that is used to promote wellness and alleviate a wide range of health conditions. Below we will discuss how to incorporate TCM principles into your acupressure practice.

The fundamental principles of TCM include the concepts of Qi, Yin and Yang, and the Five Elements. Qi, pronounced "chee," is the vital energy that flows through the body and regulates its functions. Yin and Yang represent the two opposing forces in the universe that must be in balance for optimal health. The Five Elements are wood, fire, earth, metal, and water, which represent different aspects of the body and the natural world.

Incorporating TCM principles into your acupressure practice means that you will consider these fundamental concepts and their interrelationships when treating your clients. For example, a client with a weak digestive system may have a deficiency of Qi in their stomach and spleen meridians, which can be treated by stimulating specific acupressure points along these meridians. However, TCM also recognizes that emotional stress and imbalances can impact digestion, and addressing those underlying causes may be necessary for long-term healing.

One way to incorporate TCM principles into your acupressure practice is to use the Five Element Theory. This theory recognizes that each of the Five Elements is associated with specific organs, emotions, and body parts. By understanding these associations, you can select acupressure points that address imbalances in a particular element. For example, the wood element is associated with the liver and gallbladder organs, the emotion of anger, and the tendons and ligaments in the body. If a client presents with anger issues or a sprained ankle, stimulating acupressure points along the liver and gallbladder meridians may be helpful.

Another way to incorporate TCM principles into your acupressure practice is to use the theory of Yin and Yang. This theory recognizes that the body is in a constant state of flux, and that health is maintained when Yin and Yang are in balance. For example, a client with a cold or flu may have an excess of Yin energy, which can be treated by stimulating acupressure points along the Yang meridians. On the other hand, a client with insomnia may have an excess of Yang energy, which can be treated by stimulating acupressure points along the Yin meridians.

Incorporating herbal remedies into your acupressure practice is another way to incorporate TCM principles. Many acupressure points have corresponding herbs that can be used to enhance their therapeutic effects. For example, the acupressure point PC6, located on the inner forearm, is commonly used to relieve nausea and vomiting. This point can be stimulated by applying pressure with the fingers or by using acupressure wristbands that apply constant pressure to the point. Additionally, drinking ginger tea or taking ginger supplements can enhance the effectiveness of PC6 for nausea relief.

It is essential to note that incorporating TCM principles into your acupressure practice requires an understanding of TCM theory and diagnosis. TCM diagnosis involves assessing the client's overall health, including their physical, emotional, and spiritual well-being. It is a holistic approach that takes into consideration the client's constitution, lifestyle, and environment. A TCM diagnosis can guide the selection of acupressure

Chapter Twenty-One

Acupressure for Spiritual Growth

Acupressure is a form of traditional Chinese medicine that is often used to promote physical healing and wellness. However, acupressure can also be a powerful tool for promoting spiritual growth and emotional well-being.

At its core, acupressure is based on the concept of Qi, or vital energy. According to traditional Chinese medicine, Qi flows through the body along channels known as meridians. These meridians correspond to different organs and functions of the body, and disruptions in the flow of Qi can lead to physical and emotional symptoms.

Acupressure is based on the idea that applying pressure to specific points on the body can help to balance the flow of Qi and promote healing. By stimulating these points, acupressure can help to release tension and blockages in the body, improve circulation, and support the body's natural healing processes.

But beyond its physical benefits, acupressure can also be a powerful tool for promoting spiritual growth and emotional well-being. By working with the body's energy system, acupressure can help to promote greater awareness and understanding of our own inner selves, and support us in our spiritual journeys.

One of the key ways that acupressure can support spiritual growth is by helping us to release emotional blockages and negative patterns of thought and behavior. When we experience emotional or mental distress, this can often manifest as tension or discomfort in the body. By working with specific acupressure points, we can help to release this tension and promote a greater sense of relaxation and well-being.

In addition, acupressure can help us to cultivate greater awareness and mindfulness in our daily lives. By practicing acupressure regularly, we can become more attuned to our own bodies and emotions, and develop a deeper understanding of the ways in which our thoughts and feelings impact our physical health.

One of the most powerful ways to incorporate acupressure into our spiritual practices is by working with specific points that correspond to the chakras, or energy centers of the body. In traditional Chinese medicine, there are twelve primary meridians that correspond to different organs and functions of the body, as well as several extra meridians that correspond to the chakras.

Each chakra corresponds to a different aspect of our being, and by working with specific acupressure points, we can help to balance and harmonize the energy of each chakra. This can help us to overcome emotional blockages and negative patterns of thought and behavior, and support us in our spiritual growth and development.

For example, the heart chakra is associated with love, compassion, and emotional healing. By working with specific acupressure points on the chest and upper back, we can help to release tension and blockages in this area, and promote a greater sense of openness and compassion.

Similarly, the crown chakra is associated with spiritual awareness and connection to higher consciousness. By working with acupressure points on the top of the head, we can help to release tension and blockages in this area, and promote a greater sense of spiritual connection and awareness.

Of course, as with any form of spiritual practice, it is important to approach acupressure with an open mind and a willingness to explore and experiment. There is no one "right" way to practice acupressure for spiritual growth, and different individuals may find that different techniques and approaches work best for them.

However, by working with acupressure as a tool for promoting spiritual growth and emotional well-being, we can tap into the ancient wisdom of traditional Chinese medicine and harness the power of our own bodies to support our spiritual journeys. Whether we are seeking to release emotional blockages, cultivate greater mindfulness and awareness, or deepen our connection to higher consciousness, acupressure

Balancing the Chakras

Acupressure, an ancient healing technique rooted in Traditional Chinese Medicine, is believed to balance the body's natural energy flow, or Qi. One important aspect of acupressure is the balancing of the chakras, which are seven energy centers in the body that are said to correspond to different physical, emotional, and spiritual aspects of the self. Balancing the chakras through acupressure can lead to improved overall health and spiritual growth.

To understand how acupressure can balance the chakras, it is first necessary to have a basic understanding of what the chakras are and how they function. The chakras are spinning vortexes of energy located along the spine, each associated with a different color, element, and aspect of the self. The seven chakras are the root, sacral, solar plexus, heart, throat, third eye, and crown chakras. When these chakras are balanced and aligned, energy flows freely throughout the body, promoting overall health and well-being.

Acupressure is a technique that involves applying pressure to specific points along the body's meridians, or energy pathways. By applying pressure to these points, energy blockages can be released, allowing Qi to flow freely and restoring balance to the body's systems. In the case of chakra balancing, acupressure is used to stimulate specific points associated with each of the seven chakras.

The root chakra, located at the base of the spine, is associated with grounding, stability, and survival. Acupressure points associated with the root chakra include the Bubbling Spring point on the soles of the feet, as well as points along the spine and lower back.

The sacral chakra, located just below the navel, is associated with creativity, sexuality, and pleasure. Acupressure points associated with the sacral chakra include points on the lower abdomen and inner thighs.

The solar plexus chakra, located in the upper abdomen, is associated with personal power, willpower, and confidence. Acupressure points associated with the solar plexus chakra include points on the abdomen and upper back.

The heart chakra, located in the center of the chest, is associated with love, compassion, and emotional well-being. Acupressure points associated with the heart chakra include points on the chest and upper back.

The throat chakra, located at the base of the neck, is associated with communication, self-expression, and creativity. Acupressure points associated with the throat chakra include points on the neck and shoulders.

The third eye chakra, located in the center of the forehead, is associated with intuition, perception, and spiritual awareness. Acupressure points associated with the third eye chakra include points on the forehead and temples.

The crown chakra, located at the top of the head, is associated with spiritual connection, enlightenment, and transcendence. Acupressure points associated with the crown chakra include points on the top of the head and along the midline of the body.

By applying pressure to these specific acupressure points, energy blockages can be released, allowing Qi to flow freely through the body's energy pathways and promoting balance and alignment of the chakras. In addition to acupressure, other techniques such as meditation, yoga, and aromatherapy can also be used to balance the chakras and promote spiritual growth.

Incorporating acupressure for chakra balancing into a daily self-care routine can have numerous benefits, including improved physical health, emotional stability, and spiritual growth. It is important to note that while acupressure is generally considered safe, it is always best to consult

Cultivating Inner Peace

Acupressure is a traditional Chinese medicine technique that has been used for thousands of years to promote physical, mental, and emotional health. While acupressure is often associated with relieving physical pain and discomfort, it can also be a powerful tool for cultivating inner peace and emotional balance. Below we will explore the ways in which acupressure can be used to promote inner peace and emotional wellbeing.

Acupressure works by stimulating specific points on the body known as acupoints. Each acupoint corresponds to a specific meridian, or pathway, through which vital energy, or Qi, flows. By stimulating these points, acupressure practitioners aim to rebalance the flow of energy in the body and promote healing.

One way that acupressure can promote inner peace is by calming the mind and reducing stress and anxiety. Stress is a common problem in today's fast-paced world, and can lead to a variety of physical and mental health problems. By stimulating certain acupoints, acupressure can help to activate the body's relaxation response, which in turn reduces stress and anxiety levels.

One acupoint that is particularly effective for calming the mind is known as the "Yin Tang" point. This point is located on the forehead, between the eyebrows, and is often referred to as the "Third Eye" point. By applying gentle pressure to this point, acupressure practitioners can help to relieve tension and promote a sense of inner calm.

Another acupoint that can be effective for reducing stress and anxiety is the "Heart 7" point. This point is located on the wrist, on the inside of the arm, and is said to be connected to the heart meridian. Stimulating this point with gentle pressure can help to reduce feelings of nervousness and promote a sense of calm.

In addition to promoting relaxation and reducing stress, acupressure can also be used to address deeper emotional issues. According to traditional Chinese medicine, emotions are closely linked to the body's internal organs, and imbalances in the organs can lead to emotional imbalances. By stimulating specific acupoints, acupressure practitioners can help to rebalance the internal organs and promote emotional wellbeing.

For example, the "Liver 3" acupoint is said to be connected to the liver meridian, which is associated with anger and frustration. By stimulating this point with gentle pressure, acupressure practitioners can help to release pent-up emotions and promote a sense of emotional balance.

Another acupoint that is effective for promoting emotional wellbeing is the "Pericardium 6" point. This point is located on the wrist, on the inside of the arm, and is said to be connected to the pericardium meridian, which is associated with emotional stability. Stimulating this point with gentle pressure can help to reduce anxiety and promote a sense of calm and emotional balance.

In addition to promoting relaxation and emotional balance, acupressure can also be used to promote spiritual growth and inner peace. According to traditional Chinese medicine, each meridian is associated with a specific element, such as wood, fire, earth, metal, or water. By stimulating the acupoints associated with each element, acupressure practitioners can help to balance the body's energy and promote spiritual growth.

For example, the "Kidney 1" point is associated with the water element, which is associated with wisdom and spiritual growth. By stimulating this point with gentle pressure, acupressure practitioners can help to activate the body's innate wisdom and promote spiritual growth and inner peace.

Another acupoint that is effective for promoting spiritual growth is the "Conception Vessel 17" point. This point is located on the sternum, in the

Enhancing Meditation and Mindfulness

Acupressure is an ancient healing technique that has been used for thousands of years to promote physical, emotional, and spiritual wellness. It involves applying pressure to specific points on the body to stimulate the flow of energy and promote healing. One area where acupressure can be particularly effective is in enhancing meditation and mindfulness.

Meditation is a powerful tool for reducing stress and promoting relaxation. It involves training the mind to focus on the present moment and let go of distractions and worries. Acupressure can be used to enhance the benefits of meditation by helping to release tension and promote deep relaxation.

There are several acupressure points that can be used to enhance meditation and mindfulness. The first is the third eye point, which is located between the eyebrows. This point is believed to be the center of intuition and can help to improve focus and concentration during meditation.

To stimulate the third eye point, apply gentle pressure to the area between the eyebrows using your index or middle finger. Hold the pressure for a few seconds, then release. Repeat this process several times, focusing on your breath and allowing yourself to relax.

Another acupressure point that can be used to enhance meditation is the heart point. This point is located in the center of the chest and is believed to be the center of love and compassion. Stimulating the heart point can help to promote feelings of inner peace and emotional balance.

To stimulate the heart point, place your hand over your heart and apply gentle pressure. Hold the pressure for a few seconds, then release. Repeat this process several times, focusing on your breath and allowing yourself to feel a sense of calm and relaxation.

The third acupressure point that can be used to enhance meditation is the crown point. This point is located at the top of the head and is believed to be the center of spiritual awareness. Stimulating the crown point can help to promote feelings of connection to a higher power and enhance spiritual growth.

To stimulate the crown point, use your fingertips to apply gentle pressure to the top of your head. Hold the pressure for a few seconds, then release. Repeat this process several times, allowing yourself to feel a sense of openness and connection to the universe.

In addition to these specific acupressure points, there are also general techniques that can be used to enhance meditation and mindfulness. One of these techniques is called ear massaging, which involves gently massaging the ears to stimulate the acupressure points located there.

To perform ear massaging, use your fingertips to massage the earlobes, the outer edges of the ears, and the crevices behind the ears. You can also gently pull on the earlobes and roll them between your fingers. This technique can help to release tension and promote relaxation, making it easier to focus during meditation.

Another general acupressure technique that can be used to enhance meditation is called the palm press. This technique involves pressing the palms of the hands together in front of the chest and holding the pressure for a few seconds before releasing.

To perform the palm press, sit in a comfortable position with your eyes closed and your hands resting on your knees. Take a deep breath in, then press your palms together in front of your chest as you exhale. Hold the pressure for a few seconds, then release. Repeat this process several times, focusing on your breath and allowing yourself to relax.

Chapter Twenty-Two

The Role of Nutrition in Acupressure

Acupressure is a form of traditional Chinese medicine that involves applying pressure to specific points on the body to promote healing and alleviate pain. While acupressure is often associated with the use of pressure points and massage techniques, nutrition can also play an important role in supporting the practice of acupressure.

According to traditional Chinese medicine, food is seen as a form of medicine, with certain foods believed to have specific properties that can support health and balance within the body. For example, some foods are considered to be "warming," while others are believed to be "cooling." Additionally, some foods are thought to promote circulation or support the immune system.

When incorporating acupressure into one's overall health and wellness routine, it can be helpful to consider the role of nutrition and how it may support the practice. Here are a few key considerations:

1. Choosing Nutrient-Dense Foods: In order to support overall health and wellness, it is important to choose a variety of nutrient-dense foods. This includes foods that are rich in vitamins, minerals, and antioxidants. Additionally, consuming adequate protein, healthy fats, and complex carbohydrates can help provide the body with the energy and nutrients it needs to function optimally.

2. Paying Attention to Food Energetics: Traditional Chinese medicine views food in terms of its energetics, with different foods believed to have warming, cooling, or neutral properties. When selecting foods to support acupressure, it can be helpful to choose foods that are in line with the energetics of the body and the specific goals of the acupressure practice.

3. Supporting Digestion: A healthy digestive system is essential for overall health and wellness, as it allows the body to absorb and utilize nutrients from food. When practicing acupressure, it is important to support digestion by eating a balanced diet and paying attention to digestive health. This may include consuming foods that are high in fiber, drinking plenty of water, and incorporating probiotics and other gut-supportive foods into the diet.

4. Focusing on Anti-Inflammatory Foods: Inflammation is a natural response within the body, but chronic inflammation can contribute to a wide range of health issues. When practicing acupressure, it can be helpful to focus on consuming anti-inflammatory foods, such as those that are high in omega-3 fatty acids, antioxidants, and other anti-inflammatory compounds. This may include foods like fatty fish, leafy greens, berries, and turmeric.

5. Supporting Hydration: Adequate hydration is essential for overall health and wellness, and it can also support the practice of acupressure. When practicing acupressure, it is important to drink plenty of water throughout the day to support the flow of energy throughout the body.

In addition to considering the role of nutrition in supporting acupressure, it is also important to work with a qualified acupressure practitioner who can provide guidance and support throughout the practice. A practitioner can help identify areas of the body that may benefit from acupressure, and can also recommend specific pressure points and techniques to support overall health and wellness.

Foods that Support Energy Flow

Acupressure is an ancient healing practice that involves applying pressure to specific points on the body to promote relaxation, improve circulation, and alleviate pain. In traditional Chinese medicine (TCM), acupressure is based on the concept of energy flow, or qi, which travels through the body along channels called meridians. When the flow of energy is blocked or disrupted, it can lead to physical and emotional imbalances.

One way to support the flow of energy through the body is through proper nutrition. According to TCM principles, different foods have different energetic properties that can either support or disrupt the flow of energy. Here are some foods that are believed to support energy flow and can be incorporated into a diet that complements acupressure therapy:

1. Ginger: Ginger is known for its warming and stimulating properties. It is believed to promote circulation and help ease digestive discomfort, making it a great addition to a diet that supports acupressure.

2. Garlic: Garlic has antimicrobial properties and is believed to boost the immune system. It is also said to support circulation and help regulate blood pressure, making it a valuable addition to an acupressure-focused diet.

3. Green Leafy Vegetables: Dark, leafy greens like spinach, kale, and collard greens are rich in vitamins and minerals that support overall health. They are also believed to help nourish the liver, which plays a key role in the body's detoxification process.

4. Whole Grains: Whole grains like brown rice, quinoa, and millet are a good source of complex carbohydrates, which provide sustained energy. They are also believed to support digestion and nourish the spleen, which is an important organ in TCM that is responsible for transforming food into energy.

5. Citrus Fruits: Citrus fruits like oranges, lemons, and grapefruits are rich in vitamin C, which is important for immune function and collagen production. They are also believed to help regulate qi and promote digestion.

6. Nuts and Seeds: Nuts and seeds like almonds, walnuts, and sunflower seeds are a good source of protein and healthy fats, which provide sustained energy. They are also believed to support the kidneys, which play a key role in the body's energy production and storage.

7. Fermented Foods: Fermented foods like miso, kimchi, and sauerkraut are rich in probiotics, which support digestive health and help regulate the immune system. They are also believed to support the spleen and help regulate qi.

In addition to incorporating these foods into your diet, it is also important to stay hydrated by drinking plenty of water and herbal teas. TCM principles suggest that drinking warm or room temperature liquids is better than cold liquids, as they are believed to support circulation and digestion.

It is worth noting that individual dietary needs may vary depending on factors such as age, health status, and activity level. It is always best to consult with a qualified healthcare professional, such as a registered dietitian or acupressure practitioner, to develop a personalized nutrition plan that complements your acupressure therapy.

The Importance of Hydration

The human body is composed of about 60% water, making hydration an essential part of maintaining good health. Water is responsible for transporting nutrients, regulating body temperature, and removing waste products from the body. Additionally, water is an important component of the blood, which carries oxygen and other vital substances to various organs and tissues. Dehydration can have serious consequences for our health, leading to a variety of symptoms ranging from mild to severe.

In the practice of acupressure, the importance of hydration cannot be overstated. Acupressure is a traditional Chinese medicine technique that involves applying pressure to specific points on the body to promote healing and balance. This practice is based on the concept of qi, which is the life force energy that flows through the body. When qi is flowing freely, the body is healthy and balanced. However, when qi is blocked or stagnant, health problems can arise.

One of the main goals of acupressure is to promote the free flow of qi throughout the body. This can be achieved through a variety of techniques, including applying pressure to specific acupressure points, practicing breathing exercises, and incorporating dietary and lifestyle changes.

One of the most important dietary changes that can support the free flow of qi is proper hydration. When the body is dehydrated, the flow of qi can become stagnant, leading to a variety of symptoms such as headaches, fatigue, and digestive problems. By staying hydrated, we can support the free flow of qi and promote overall health and well-being.

In addition to drinking plenty of water, there are certain foods and beverages that can support hydration and the flow of qi. These include:

1. Water-rich fruits and vegetables: Fruits and vegetables that are high in water content, such as cucumbers, watermelon, and celery, can help to support hydration and promote the free flow of qi.

2. Herbal teas: Herbal teas such as peppermint, ginger, and chamomile can help to support hydration and promote the free flow of qi.

3. Electrolyte-rich drinks: Drinks that contain electrolytes, such as coconut water or sports drinks, can help to support hydration and promote the free flow of qi.

4. Warm fluids: Drinking warm fluids, such as warm water or herbal teas, can help to support the free flow of qi and promote overall health and well-being.

It is also important to be mindful of factors that can contribute to dehydration, such as excessive sweating, caffeine and alcohol consumption, and certain medications. When practicing acupressure, it is important to stay hydrated and avoid these dehydrating factors as much as possible.

In addition to supporting hydration, acupressure can also be used to promote the free flow of qi and support overall health and well-being. By incorporating acupressure techniques into our daily routine and staying hydrated, we can promote the flow of qi and support our body's natural healing processes.

Dietary Considerations for Optimal Results

Acupressure is an ancient healing practice that has been used for thousands of years to promote health and well-being. It is based on the principles of traditional Chinese medicine and involves the application of pressure to specific points on the body. While acupressure can be a powerful tool for healing, it is important to remember that it is just one aspect of a holistic approach to health. Along with acupressure, dietary considerations can play a significant role in achieving optimal results.

In traditional Chinese medicine, food is considered to be medicine. What we eat can either support or hinder our health, depending on our choices. According to TCM principles, certain foods have specific properties that can either cool or warm the body, nourish specific organs, and affect energy flow. By choosing foods that support our unique needs, we can help to balance our bodies and promote optimal health.

One of the most important dietary considerations in TCM is maintaining balance. This means eating a balanced diet of whole, natural foods that provide a variety of nutrients. In TCM, it is believed that each organ has a specific flavor that nourishes it. For example, the liver is nourished by sour flavors, the spleen by sweet flavors, and the heart by bitter flavors. By including a variety of flavors in our diet, we can help to ensure that all of our organs are properly nourished.

Another important consideration is eating foods that are in season. According to TCM, each season has a specific energy that affects the body. By eating foods that are in season, we can help to balance our bodies with the energy of the season. For example, in the summer, it is important to eat cooling foods like watermelon, cucumber, and mint to help balance the heat of the season.

In TCM, it is also believed that the digestive system plays a key role in overall health. When the digestive system is functioning properly, the body is better able to absorb nutrients and eliminate waste. To support digestion, it is important to eat slowly and mindfully, chew food thoroughly, and avoid overeating. Eating warm, cooked foods is also beneficial for digestion, as they are easier to digest than raw foods.

When it comes to acupressure, dietary considerations can also play a role in promoting optimal results. For example, if someone is experiencing digestive issues, acupressure points on the stomach and large intestine meridians may be used to help stimulate digestion. In addition, acupressure points on the spleen and liver meridians may be used to help support the body's ability to absorb nutrients.

Incorporating certain foods into the diet can also be beneficial when combined with acupressure. For example, ginger is a common ingredient in TCM that is believed to help stimulate digestion, reduce inflammation, and support the immune system. By incorporating ginger into the diet and using acupressure points on the stomach and spleen meridians, digestive issues may be addressed more effectively.

Chapter Twenty-Three

The Power of Touch

The power of touch is an essential part of human connection and communication. From a simple hug to a massage, touch has been shown to have a significant impact on our physical and emotional well-being. Acupressure is a form of touch therapy that involves applying pressure to specific points on the body to stimulate the body's natural healing processes. This ancient technique has been used for thousands of years and is still widely practiced today.

Acupressure is based on the same principles as acupuncture, which is an ancient Chinese practice that involves inserting thin needles into specific points on the body to promote healing. Acupressure, on the other hand, uses fingers, hands, or other tools to apply pressure to the same points. These pressure points are believed to be connected to various organs and systems in the body and, by stimulating them, can help to relieve pain, reduce stress, and improve overall health and well-being.

One of the primary benefits of acupressure is its ability to promote relaxation and reduce stress. Stress is a leading cause of many health problems, including anxiety, depression, and heart disease. By stimulating specific pressure points, acupressure can help to activate the body's natural relaxation response, which can reduce stress levels and promote a sense of calm and well-being.

Acupressure has also been shown to be effective in relieving pain. By stimulating specific pressure points, acupressure can help to reduce inflammation and improve blood flow to the affected area, which can reduce pain and promote healing. It has been used to relieve pain associated with conditions such as arthritis, headaches, and menstrual cramps.

In addition to its physical benefits, acupressure is also believed to have emotional and spiritual benefits. According to traditional Chinese medicine, each pressure point is connected to a specific emotion, and stimulating these points can help to balance emotions and promote emotional well-being. For example, the pressure point located between the eyebrows is believed to be connected to the emotion of worry. Stimulating this point may help to reduce feelings of anxiety and promote a sense of calm.

There are many different techniques and styles of acupressure, each with its own unique benefits and applications. Some practitioners use finger pressure, while others use tools such as rollers or acupressure mats. Some techniques involve gentle pressure, while others use more forceful pressure or stretching. The key to effective acupressure is finding the right pressure points and applying the right amount of pressure to achieve the desired result.

Acupressure can be practiced by anyone and can be performed on oneself or on others. It is often used in conjunction with other therapies, such as massage, yoga, or acupuncture. While it is generally considered safe, it is important to consult with a qualified practitioner before beginning any new therapy or treatment.

The Healing Potential of Human Connection

Acupressure is an ancient healing technique that has been used for thousands of years to promote physical and emotional well-being. The practice involves the application of pressure to specific points on the body, known as acupoints, which are believed to be connected to various organs and systems of the body. Acupressure is a form of touch therapy that not only promotes physical healing but also provides emotional support and promotes human connection.

Human connection is essential for our physical and emotional well-being. When we are connected to others, we experience a sense of belonging, comfort, and security. The power of touch is a fundamental aspect of human connection, and it has been shown to have many positive effects on the body and mind. Studies have shown that touch therapy can help reduce stress, anxiety, and depression, improve immune function, and promote relaxation.

Acupressure takes the power of touch to a whole new level. By applying pressure to specific acupoints, acupressure practitioners can stimulate the body's natural healing processes and promote a sense of well-being. This technique is particularly effective for conditions related to stress, anxiety, and pain. It is also used to promote relaxation, improve sleep, and boost the immune system.

One of the most significant benefits of acupressure is its ability to promote human connection. The practice of acupressure requires the practitioner to be in close contact with the client, often using their hands to apply pressure to various acupoints on the body. This physical contact can help to create a sense of connection and trust between the practitioner and client, which can be especially important for individuals who are experiencing emotional distress.

Studies have shown that touch therapy, such as acupressure, can increase levels of oxytocin in the body. Oxytocin is a hormone that is associated with social bonding and emotional attachment. When levels of oxytocin are increased, individuals may experience a greater sense of trust, connection, and emotional well-being.

In addition to promoting human connection, acupressure can also be used to enhance other forms of therapy. For example, acupressure can be used in combination with talk therapy to help individuals work through emotional issues. By promoting relaxation and reducing stress, acupressure can help individuals to feel more comfortable and open during therapy sessions, making it easier to explore and address emotional issues.

Acupressure can also be used in conjunction with other forms of complementary and alternative medicine, such as acupuncture and herbal medicine. When used together, these modalities can provide a holistic approach to healing that addresses not only physical symptoms but also emotional and spiritual well-being.

Building Trust and Rapport with Clients

Acupressure is a form of alternative medicine that uses pressure on specific points on the body to help relieve pain and tension, improve circulation, and promote relaxation. A successful acupressure practice not only requires the technical skills to perform the therapy effectively, but also the ability to build trust and rapport with clients.

Building trust and rapport with clients is essential in any healthcare practice, but it is particularly important in acupressure, as the practice involves physical contact and requires clients to be open and vulnerable. One way to build trust is to create a safe and welcoming environment. This can be achieved by maintaining a clean and organized workspace, providing comfortable seating or a massage table, and using soothing scents or soft lighting to create a calming atmosphere.

It is also important to communicate clearly and effectively with clients. This means explaining the acupressure process, including what to expect during the session, and answering any questions or concerns the client may have. Practitioners should also take the time to listen to clients' concerns and goals, as well as any feedback they may have about the session.

In addition, practitioners should always obtain informed consent from clients before beginning any acupressure session. This means explaining the risks and benefits of the therapy, as well as any potential side effects or contraindications. Clients should also be given the opportunity to ask questions and voice any concerns they may have before giving their consent.

Another key aspect of building trust and rapport with clients is developing a strong sense of empathy. Practitioners should strive to understand and relate to clients' experiences and emotions, and provide a safe and supportive space for them to express their feelings. This can be achieved through active listening, validating clients' feelings, and providing emotional support as needed.

It is also important for practitioners to be transparent and honest with clients. This means being upfront about fees and payment policies, as well as any limitations or qualifications of the practitioner. Clients should be informed of any potential conflicts of interest, such as selling products or services, and given the option to decline any additional offerings.

To build a successful acupressure practice, practitioners must also be knowledgeable about the therapy and its benefits. This includes staying up to date with current research and developments in the field, as well as attending trainings and workshops to improve their skills and knowledge. By staying informed and knowledgeable, practitioners can provide the best possible care for their clients and build trust in their abilities.

The Impact of Touch on Emotional Well-being

The sense of touch is one of the most powerful senses we possess. It is through touch that we connect with the world around us and with others. Acupressure is an ancient healing technique that utilizes touch to promote physical, emotional, and mental well-being. It is based on the idea that energy flows through the body along specific pathways or meridians, and that by applying pressure to specific points along these pathways, the flow of energy can be restored and balanced.

Acupressure has been found to have a significant impact on emotional well-being. Many of the acupressure points are located on or near the major nerve centers of the body. By stimulating these points, the nervous system is activated, releasing neurotransmitters such as endorphins and serotonin, which are associated with feelings of happiness, relaxation, and well-being. This can be particularly helpful for those struggling with anxiety, depression, or other emotional disorders.

One of the most significant benefits of acupressure for emotional well-being is its ability to reduce stress. Stress is a common problem in today's fast-paced world, and it can have a significant impact on both physical and emotional health. Chronic stress can lead to anxiety, depression, and a weakened immune system, making it more difficult for the body to fight off illness and disease.

Acupressure has been found to be an effective way to reduce stress and promote relaxation. By stimulating specific points on the body, acupressure can help to reduce tension in the muscles, lower blood pressure, and slow down the heart rate. This can lead to a feeling of calm and relaxation, which can help to reduce feelings of anxiety and stress.

Acupressure can also be helpful for those struggling with addiction. Addiction is often a result of a lack of emotional balance, and acupressure can help to restore balance to the body and mind. By stimulating specific points on the body, acupressure can help to reduce cravings, promote relaxation, and increase feelings of well-being. This can be particularly helpful for those in recovery from addiction, as it can help to reduce the risk of relapse.

Another way that acupressure can impact emotional well-being is through its ability to promote better sleep. Many people struggle with sleep problems, which can be caused by a variety of factors, including stress, anxiety, and physical discomfort. Acupressure can help to promote relaxation, reduce stress, and alleviate physical discomfort, all of which can lead to a better night's sleep. Better sleep can lead to improved emotional health, as it can help to reduce feelings of fatigue and irritability.

Acupressure can also be helpful for those dealing with grief and loss. The emotional pain of grief can be overwhelming, and it can be difficult to know how to cope with these feelings. Acupressure can help to promote emotional healing by stimulating the body's natural healing mechanisms. By promoting relaxation and reducing stress, acupressure can help to reduce feelings of sadness and promote a sense of peace.

9781776968206
SD - #0164 - 070926 - C0 - 229/152/11 - PB - 9781776968206 - Matt Lamination